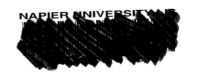

A Colour Handbook of

HEART FAILURE

Investigation, Diagnosis, Treatment

MICHAEL D SOSIN
Specialist Registrar in Cardiology
Department of Cardiology,
Queen's Medical Centre, Nottingham

GURBIR BHATIA
Specialist Registrar in Cardiology
Department of Cardiology,
City General Hospital, Stoke on Trent, UK

GREGORY YH LIP
Professor of Cardiovascular Medicine
University Department of Medicine,
City Hospital, Birmingham, UK

MICHAEL K DAVIES
Consultant Cardiologist
The Queen Elizabeth Hospital, Birmingham, UK

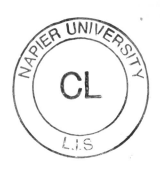
MANSON
PUBLISHING

Abbreviations

ACE	angiotensin-converting enzyme		JVP	jugular venous pulsation
ADH	antidiuretic hormone		LV	left ventricle/left ventricular
AF	atrial fibrillation		LVD	left ventricular dysfunction
AMP	adenosine monophosphate		LVEDV	left ventricular end-diastolic volume
ANP	atrial natriuretic peptide		LVEF	left ventricular ejection fraction
ARB	angiotensin II receptor blocker		MI	myocardial infarction
BNP	brain natriuretic peptide		MMP	matrix metalloproteinase
CAD	coronary artery disease		MUGA	multi-gated ventriculography
CNP	C-type natriuretic peptide		NEP	neutral endopeptidase
CO	cardiac output		NICE	National Institute for Clinical Excellence
CTR	cardiothoracic ratio		NO	nitric oxide
ECG	electrocardiogram		NOS	nitric oxide synthase
ECM	extracellular matrix		NSAID	nonsteroidal anti-inflammatory drug
ET	endothelin		NYHA	New York Heart Association
FBC	full blood count		PND	paroxysmal nocturnal dyspnoea
GFR	glomerular filtration rate		RAAS	renin–angiotensin–aldosterone system
GMP	guanosine monophosphate		SDNN	standard deviation of R-R intervals
GTN	glyceryl trinitrate		SR	sinus rhythm
HF	heart failure		SVR	systemic vascular resistance
HIV	human immunodeficiency virus		TIMP	tissue inhibitor metalloproteinase
HR	hazard ratio		TNF	tumour necrosis factor
HRV	heart rate variability		VE	ventricular extrasystole
ICD	implantable cardioverter defibrillator		VO_2	peak oxygen uptake
ISDN	isosorbide dinitrate			

Note: Medicine is an ever-changing subject. While the authors have taken every effort to eliminate inaccuracies, readers are advised to check recommended doses in the drug data sheets before prescribing regimens. Drug licensing varies from country to country; the information given in this book mainly reflects UK practice.

Copyright © 2006 Manson Publishing Ltd

ISBN 1–84076–059–1
ISBN 978–1–84076–059–0

A CIP catalogue record for this book is available from the British Library.

For full details of all Manson Publishing Ltd titles please write to:
Manson Publishing Ltd, 73 Corringham Road, London NW11 7DL, UK.
Tel: +44(0)20 8905 5150
Fax: +44(0)20 8201 9233
Website: www.mansonpublishing.com

Commissioning editor: Jill Northcott
Project manager: Paul Bennett
Copy-editor: Ruth Maxwell
Cover and book design: Cathy Martin, Presspack Computing Ltd
Illustrations and layout: Cathy Martin, Presspack Computing Ltd
Colour reproduction: Tenon & Polert Colour Scanning Ltd, Hong Kong
Printed by: Grafos SA, Barcelona, Spain

Contents

Preface

Heart failure is a disease with stark implications: a markedly reduced life expectancy and diminished quality of life. Heart failure is the only area of cardiovascular medicine in which the disease burden is rising in the western world, with an estimated lifetime risk of 1 in 5. It is only in recent years that widespread recognition of these realities has generated increased interest in research in all aspects of heart failure, leading to the development of a variety of diagnostic and therapeutic modalities.

This colour handbook has been designed for those seeking a comprehensive overview of all aspects of heart failure. This highly illustrated handbook is organized into chapters, each focussing on a different area of heart failure management, starting with epidemiological background, moving through a description of the classical clinical features of the disease, and providing a summary of available diagnostic approaches. Further chapters focus on individual therapeutic options, presenting the evidence relating to the use of each in patients with heart failure. The emphasis of treatment in heart failure may also be shifting toward nondrug management, including specialist heart failure nursing and device therapy. The importance of effective palliative care cannot be overestimated as patients may value quality over quantity of life; all of these subjects are addressed. As evidence of the ongoing research effort in heart failure, the final chapter describes exciting new approaches and technologies which might, in the future, make a real difference to patients with this devastating condition.

The main feature of this handbook is that all chapters are fully illustrated, with information from landmark trials, patient photographs, cardiological investigations, and examples of the many imaging modalities used in the management of patients with heart failure.

We hope that this book will both inform and encourage all those who participate in the care of patients with heart failure

Michael D Sosin
Gurbir Bhatia
Gregory YH Lip
Michael K Davies

Chapter one

Epidemiology

What is heart failure?

Heart failure (HF) is a common syndrome resulting from a variety of cardiac diseases and is characterized by a reduced cardiac output that is unable to meet the metabolic needs of the body. It is a major cause of morbidity and mortality, and places a considerable economic burden upon health-care institutions. The prevalence and cost of management are likely to rise in the future as the population is ageing, and is being exposed to improved treatment (and improved subsequent survival) of myocardial infarction (MI).

In the past, assessment of the epidemiology of HF has been problematic due to difficulties in its diagnosis. For example, clinical signs are not specific to HF, and may result from other common medical conditions. Furthermore, studies investigating HF have not employed a consistent definition of heart failure, making comparisons difficult. In the last decade, the European Society of Cardiology (Task Force on Heart Failure) issued diagnostic guidelines (*Table 1*), which required both the presence of appropriate symptoms and objective evidence of cardiac dysfunction. Typical symptoms include dyspnoea, effort intolerance, and peripheral oedema. In cases of doubt, treatment of HF should result in symptomatic improvement.

SYSTOLIC HEART FAILURE

As outlined above, the diagnosis of HF requires objective evidence of cardiac dysfunction. Dysfunction may reflect impairment of either contractility (systolic dysfunction) or filling (diastolic dysfunction). Existing parameters to define left ventricular systolic dysfunction include assessment of ejection fraction (LVEF) and/or echocardiographic fractional shortening. LVEF <40% or fractional shortening <25% represents significant contractile impairment, and the presence of appropriate symptoms in this setting would confer a diagnosis of systolic HF (**1–3**).

DIASTOLIC HEART FAILURE

What constitutes a diagnosis of diastolic HF is less clear. A significant proportion of patients with HF appear to have preserved systolic function. Some

---

Table 1 European Society of Cardiology Diagnostic Criteria for Heart Failure

✧ Appropriate symptoms of heart failure*
✧ Objective evidence of cardiac dysfunction* (echo most practical tool)
✧ In cases of doubt, symptom improvement with heart failure therapy

These features are compulsory

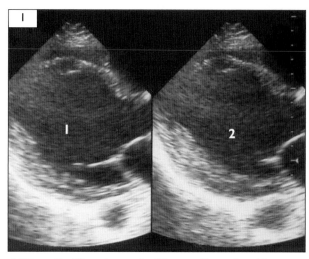

1 Diastolic (1) and systolic (2) two dimensional long axis echocardiogram from a patient with severe left ventricular dysfunction (ejection fraction 20%).

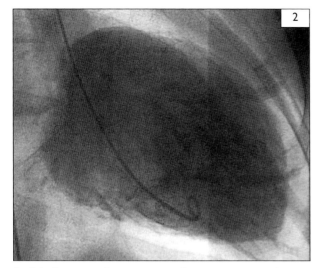
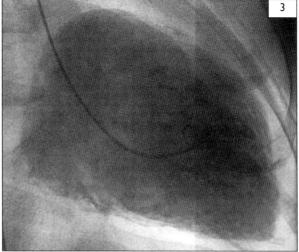

2, 3 Left ventricular angiogram from a patient with a dilated cardiomyopathy. Contractility is markedly reduced with the systolic (**2**) and diastolic (**3**) frames of almost identical area.

physicians argue that certain features suggesting diastolic dysfunction need to be identified, in addition to the presence of clinical evidence of HF and demonstration of preserved (or minimally reduced) LVEF. Diastolic indices relating to ventricular filling, relaxation, distensibility, or stiffness may be assessed (e.g. by echocardiography), although such parameters vary with age and standardization is difficult. Other physicians, however, suggest that diastolic HF may be diagnosed without assessment of diastolic indices, and merely requires the presence of symptoms with retained systolic function.

The scope of the problem

Several epidemiological studies of HF have been performed in the last half-century. The most well known is the Framingham Heart Study. This cohort of >5000 American subjects was set up over 50 years ago, and individuals underwent clinical, electro-cardiographic, and radiographic assessment at baseline and every 2 years thereafter. The offspring of participants were added to the total pool in 1971. Thus, this is a large, prospective, and very important database. Of note, the diagnosis of heart failure in the Framingham study was made clinically, and without an objective assessment of ventricular function. Other studies have included echocardio-graphic analysis of ventricular function in detailing the prevalence of HF. For example, the ECHOES study group has investigated the prevalence of HF and left ventricular systolic dysfunction in nearly 4000 community-based subjects in the West Midlands, UK.

Table 2 Incidence and prevalence of heart failure-effect of age and gender

Age	Incidence (%)		Prevalence (%)	
	men	women	men	women
<65 years	0.1	0.04	0.1	0.1
>65 years	1.1	0.5	4	3

INCIDENCE

Estimates of the incidence of HF vary with the populations studied and the definition of HF employed. The incidence among males and females under 65 years of age is 0.1% and 0.04%, respectively, and increasing age and male gender are associated with higher incidences (*Table 2*). Indeed, Framingham data have revealed a doubling in incidence of HF with each decade of ageing. More recent analysis of the same data has shown that among males, the incidence of HF has remained essentially unchanged over the last four decades. Improved survival following MI may be responsible for the absence of a fall in incident cases in men. In contrast, the trend in incidence among females over the same time period is downward. A possible explanation may be that HF risk in females may be mainly associated with hypertension as opposed to coronary disease, which is the principal risk factor in males. Improved hypertensive control may, therefore, have resulted in the fall in incidence among females. Improved physician awareness of HF may also contribute to an increase in reported incidence.

PREVALENCE

Prevalence of HF is similarly variable and is related to study methods. Nevertheless, prevalence also rises with age (*Table 3*). Asymptomatic left ventricular systolic dysfunction has a prevalence of around 3%, and was found to be more common among men in the Glasgow MONICA survey. This asymptomatic group has lower mortality compared to those with symptoms, but still represents an important group which may benefit from treatment strategies to delay progression to HF.

The prevalence of diastolic heart failure is not clear. Recent community-based studies have suggested that >50% of prevalent cases of HF occur despite preserved systolic function. The very elderly appear to be particularly susceptible to HF in this setting. A German echocardiographic survey of a community population of >1000 subjects revealed a prevalence of diastolic abnormalities of 11%, with diastolic dysfunction found in 3.1%. Systolic dysfunction (defined by LVEF <45%) was found in 2.3%.

Who is at risk?

Longitudinal studies such as the Framingham Heart Study provide data relating to aetiologies of HF, and their respective contributions at different time periods. Such data are augmented by those obtained from large therapeutic trials.

UNDERLYING AETIOLOGY

In the 'developed' world, coronary artery disease (CAD) and hypertension are the principal aetiologies in the development of HF (*Table 4*). In the initial cohort of the Framingham study, hypertension appeared to be the most common underlying condition. However, as time progressed, an increase in the contribution of CAD (at the expense of hypertension and valvular heart disease) was noted.

CAD (**4–12**) accounts for 60–70% of cases of HF. It may contribute either by causing myocardial necrosis following infarction, or by causing resting contractile dysfunction of viable myocardium. Such dysfunction may persist after transient episodes of ischaemia (myocardial stunning) or may have the potential to recover following revascularization (hibernating myocardium).

Table 3 Prevalence of left ventricular dysfunction north Glasgow MONICA survey

Age	Asymptomatic		Symptomatic	
	men	women	men	women
45–54	4.4	1.2	1.4	1.2
55–64	3.2	0	2.5	2.0
65–74	3.2	1.3	3.2	3.6

(From McDonagh TA, *et al. Lancet* 1997;**350**:829–833.)

Table 4 Underlying aetiologies of heart failiure

Coronary artery disease (60–70%*)
◇ Myocardial infarction
◇ Myocardial hibernation or stunning

Hypertension

Cardiomyopathy
◇ Dilated e.g. idiopathic, viral myocarditis, HIV, toxins (alcohol and anthracyclines), peripartum
◇ Hypertrophic
◇ Restrictive e.g. amyloides, sarcoidosis

Valvular heart disease
◇ Mitral regurgitation
◇ Aortic stenosis

Arrhythmias

Pericardial disease (constrictive or effusive)

Congenital heart disease

*This estimate derived from information from participants of various clinical trials, with the majority of subjects male, Caucasian and aged <70 years

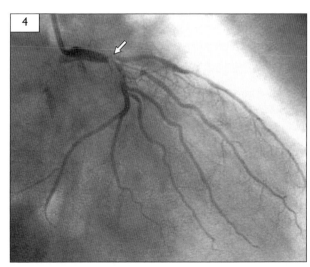

4 Coronary angiogram showing severe distal left main stem disease (arrow).

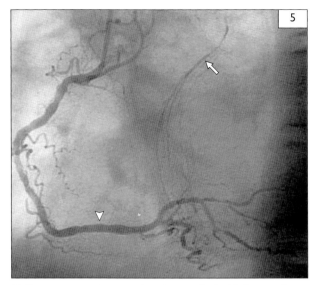

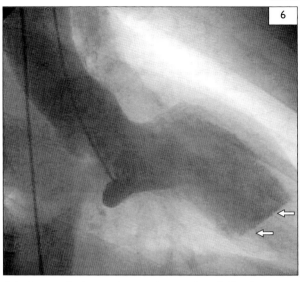

5 Coronary angiogram showing occluded left anterior descending artery (arrow) cross-filling from an injection into a diseased right coronary artery (arrowhead).

6 Left ventricular angiogram in a patient following anterior myocardial infarction showing a significant area of regional wall akinesia and dilatation together with a left ventricular thrombus (arrows).

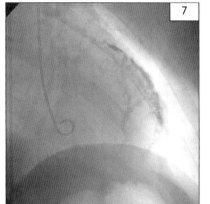

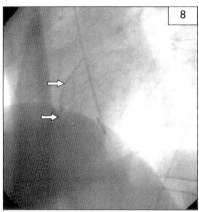

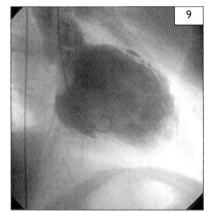

7–9 Calcified left ventricular infarct/aneurysm at cardiac catheterization RAO view (**7**), LAO view (**8**) (arrows), and on left ventricular angiography (**9**).

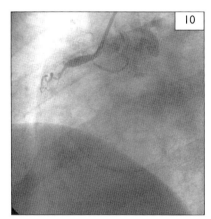

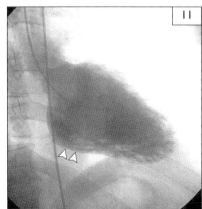

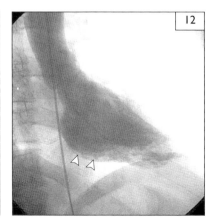

10–12 Occluded right coronary artery (**10**) subtending a large area of inferior akinesia on left ventricular angiography. Diastolic frame (**11**) and systolic frame (**12**) (arrowheads).

Hypertension, either alone or in combination with other causes, has been shown to be associated with HF in several studies, including the Framingham study (*Table 5*). Clearly, this is a risk factor for CAD itself, but may also lead to the development of HF by inducing left ventricular hypertrophy (13) or the development of atrial fibrillation (AF).

Other significant causes include idiopathic dilated cardiomyopathy (14, 15), hypertrophic (16, 17) and restrictive (18–20) cardiomyopathies, and

Table 5 Progression from hypertension to heart failure (Framingham Study)		
Total number of examinees	5143	
Number (%) developing HF	392 (7.6)	
No hypertension	35	
BP >140/90 mmHg (18.7/12 kPa)	357 (91.1%)	
	Characteristics of hypertensives prior to HF	
	Male (%)	Female (%)
BP 140–159/90–99 mmHg (18.7–21.2/12–13.2 kPa)	24	18
BP >160/100 mmHg (21.3/13.3 kPa) or on treatment	76	82
Myocardial infraction	52	34
Angina (no infarction)	12	21
Diabetes	24	28
LVH	21	23
Valvular disease	24	33

BP: blood pressure; HF: heart failure; LVH: left ventricular hypertrophy. (From Levy D, et al. JAMA 1996; **275**:1557–1562.)

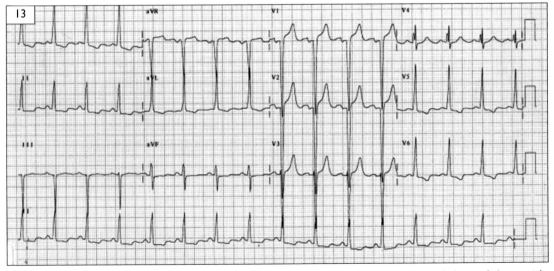

13 Electrocardiogram showing left ventricular hypertrophy in an elderly female with heart failure, with underlying hypertension and coronary artery disease.

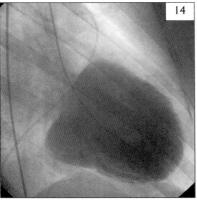

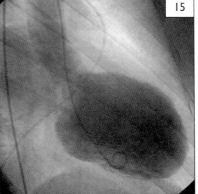

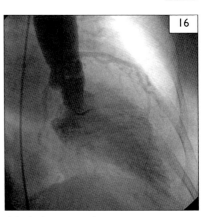

14, 15 Left ventricular angiogram diastolic frame (**14**) and systolic frame (**15**) from a patient with an idiopathic dilated cardiomyopathy.

16 Left ventricular angiogram, diastolic frame, in a patient with hypertrophic cardiomyopathy.

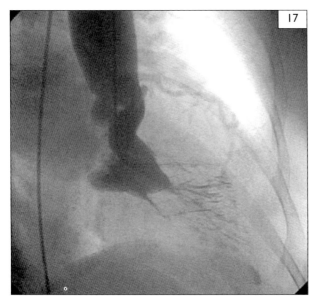

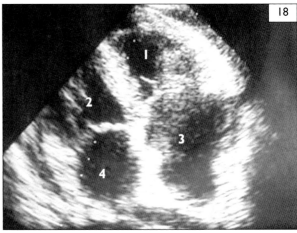

18 Amyloid heart disease as a cause of a restrictive cardiomyopathy. 2D echocardiogram showing pseudohypertrophy of the interventricular septum, right ventricular wall, and interatrial septum due to amyloid deposit. 1: right ventricle; 2: left ventricle; 3: right atrium; 4: left atrium.

17 Left ventricular angiogram, systolic frame, in hypertrophic cardiomyopathy showing apical and mid left ventricular cavity obliteration, trapping of contrast in the left ventricular apex, and some associated mitral regurgitation.

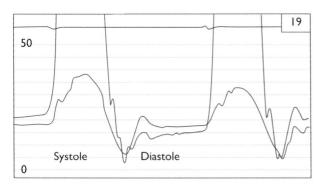

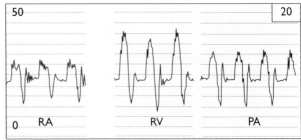

19, 20 Cardiac catheterization data in restrictive cardiomyopathy due to amyloid, showing near equalization of all cardiac diastolic pressures. **19**: equalization of right and left ventricular diastolic pressures with dip and plateau ('square root') configuration; **20**: equalization of right atrial (RA), right ventricular (RV), and pulmonary artery (PA) diastolic pressures.

valvular heart disease, such as mitral valve disease (**21–25**) and aortic valve disease (**26–33**). Of course, certain aetiologies may coexist, and the exact contribution of each to the subsequent development of HF can be unclear. An American survey of 1200 patients undergoing myocardial biopsy for initially unexplained HF, revealed that 50% of cases were due to an idiopathic cardiomyopathy. Other causes included myocarditis (9%), ischaemic heart disease

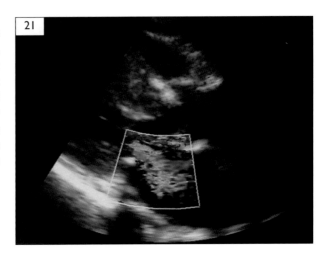

21 Moderate mitral regurgitation on colour flow Doppler.

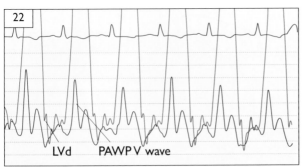

22 Moderate mitral regurgitation at cardiac catheterization – simultaneous left ventricular diastolic (LVd) and pumonary artery wedge pressure (PAWP). Large V wave in pulmonary artery wedge pressure.

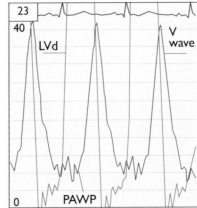

23 Severe mitral regurgitation at cardiac catheterization – simultaneous left ventricular diastolic (LVd) and pulmonary artery wedge pressure (PAWP). Large V wave >40 mmHg (5.3 kPa).

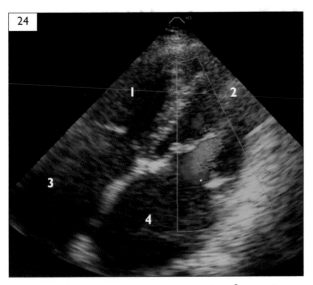

24 Mitral stenosis, mitral valve area 1.1 cm^2 on colour flow Doppler. 1: right ventricle; 2: left ventricle; 3: right atrium; 4: left atrium.

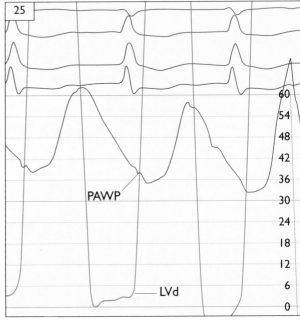

25 Severe mitral stenosis at cardiac catheterization – simultaneous left ventricular end diastolic (LVd) and pulmonary artery wedge pressure (PAWP). End-diastolic gradient approximately 30 mmHg (4 kPa).

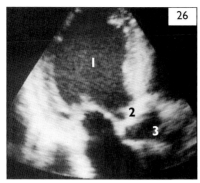

26 Two-dimensional echocardiogram in severe aortic stenosis showing a heavily calcified aortic valve and significant left ventricular hypertrophy. 1: left ventricle; 2: aortic valve; 3: aorta.

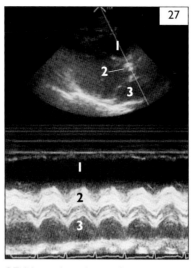

27 M-mode echocardiogram across aortic valve (long axis view) showing a heavily calcified valve with restricted opening. 1: right ventricle; 2: aortic valve; 3: left atrium.

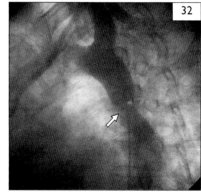

28 Cardiac catheterization data in severe aortic stenosis – simultaneous left ventricular and aortic systolic pressures. Gradient 120 mmHg (16 kPa).

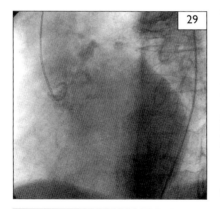

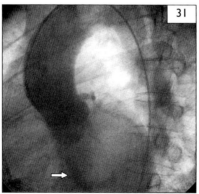

31, 32 Bicuspid aortic valve with aortic regurgitation (**31**, arrow) and coarctation of the aorta (**32**, arrow).

33 Coarctation of the aorta – simultaneous ascending aorta and femoral artery pressures. Gradient 60 mmHg (8 kPa).

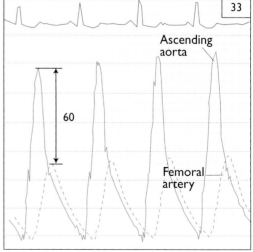

29, 30 Mixed aortic valve disease. Calcified aortic valve (**29**) and moderate to severe aortic regurgitation on aortography (**30**).

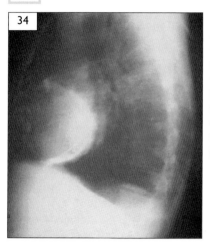

34 Lateral chest X-ray showing extensive pericardial calcification in a patient with severe peripheral oedema due to constrictive pericarditis.

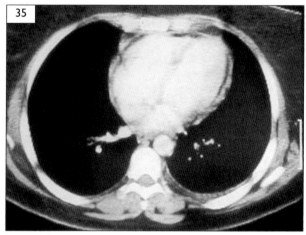

35 Computed tomography scan showing a thickened pericardium in constrictive pericarditis.

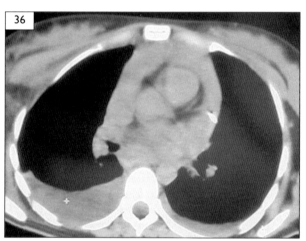

36 Computed tomography scan showing a markedly thickened pericardium due to previous purulent pericarditis.

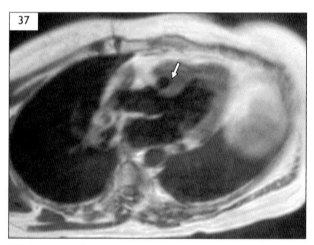

37 Computed tomography scan showing extensive endomyocardial fibrosis and near obliteration of the right ventricular cavity (arrow) due to hypereosinophilic syndrome.

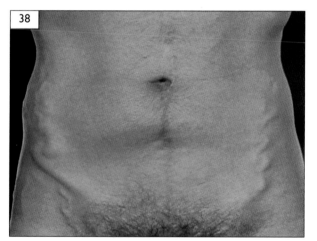

38 A case of low output cardiac failure due to inferior vena caval obstruction/ligation for previous lymphoma, showing marked venous collaterals.

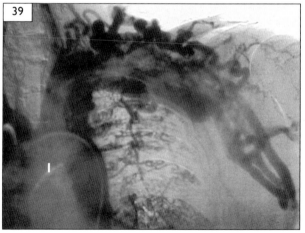

39 High output cardiac failure secondary to a subclavian arteriovenous fistula following a stab wound. 1: aorta.

(7%), and infiltrative and hypertensive heart disease (each 4%). Rare causes of HF are illustrated in **34–39**.

RISK OF DEVELOPING HEART FAILURE

Assessment of Framingham data has enabled estimates of overall risk of developing HF to be calculated (*Table 6*). After studying 8000 subjects between 1971 and 1996, lifetime risk for HF was 1 in 5, irrespective of gender. Stratification of risk by blood pressure revealed that higher blood pressure values were associated with twice the risk compared with those with lower values, again regardless of gender. However, the risks in males and females without previous MI were 1 in 9 and 1 in 6, respectively. This indicates that MI plays a greater contributory role in HF development in males than in females, in whom hypertension may be the more important factor.

Parameters that appear to confer risk of subsequent development of HF have been identified as left ventricular hypertrophy (independent of hypertension), cigarette smoking, hyperlipidaemia, and diabetes mellitus. The relative risks of these factors are higher in those <65 years, highlighting the need for risk assessment strategies in the middle-aged, rather than only in the elderly. Of course, these also represent risk factors for the development of CAD, the most common cause of HF in the west. Of note, electrocardiographic evidence of left ventricular hypertrophy (**13**) is a risk factor independent of any underlying hypertension.

EFFECT OF ETHNICITY

It should be noted that the Framingham cohort is largely Caucasian, and therefore may not be truly representative of the American (or other) populations. The relative importance of HF aetiologies may vary between different ethnic groups. For example, hypertension may be responsible for up to 50% of heart failure in African-Americans. The relative frequency of different HF aetiologies among other ethnic groups has been only minimally studied.

HEART FAILURE IN THE 'DEVELOPING' WORLD

Logistical problems in the accurate accumulation of population-based epidemiological data relating to HF in the developing world limits available information. However, hospital-based studies enable certain features to be drawn out. For example, rheumatic heart disease remains a major cause of HF in most countries. Other infective causes include Chagas' disease, which remains a significant aetiology in South America. Hypertension and CAD as underlying

Table 6 Lifetime risk of developing heart failure		
	Male	**Female**
Overall lifetime risk	20%	20%
Lifetime risk (no prior MI)	11%	16%
MI: myocardial infarction. (Adapted from Lloyd-Jones DM, *et al. Circulation* 2002;**106**: 3068.)		

diseases are not confined to the west, however, and the relative contribution of these 'western' conditions is likely to increase, resulting in greater overall cardio-vascular disease burden in these regions.

Morbidity and quality of life

Patients with HF are burdened not only by symptoms such as dyspnoea, fatigue, and peripheral oedema, but have high prevalence of comorbidities including angina, hypertension, diabetes, AF, and chronic pulmonary disease. Furthermore, patients with HF are at higher risk of developing thromboembolic complications including stroke, MI, and venous thromboembolism.

Clearly, therefore, patients with HF are likely to be dependent on frequent consultations with health-care services, in both primary care and hospital settings. HF is responsible for >5% of adult medical admissions in the UK, with admissions often lengthy, and discharge frequently followed by readmission. For example, in one study 16% of American admissions for first episodes of HF were readmitted within 6 months. Furthermore, many patients with HF require support out of hospital, ranging from social service support at home to nursing home placement. Such dependence, therefore, exemplifies the demand HF places on health-care resources.

HF has a significant, detrimental effect upon quality of life. This concept encompasses both physical and psychological wellbeing, as well as social functioning. Questionnaires to evaluate patients' perception of their quality of life have been developed, and examples include the Minnesota Living with Heart Failure questionnaire, and the SF-36 questionnaire, which is not specific to any particular condition. The ECHOES study investigators conducted a prospective evaluation of quality of life in HF patients in the community. HF was associated with reduction in physical and mental health scores, with correlation between SF-36 score and severity of HF. Physical impairment of quality of life resulting from HF exceeded that resulting from both arthritis and chronic pulmonary diseases.

Prognosis

HF is associated with a very poor prognosis, with 5-year mortality levels of up to 75%. Increasing severity of HF, older age, and male gender are associated with a worse outlook (*Table 7*). One-third of all deaths appear to be preceded by a major ischaemic event, and acute MI is associated with an eightfold increase in the risk of death. Deaths among patients with HF are frequently sudden, with Framingham data revealing a fivefold increase in risk. The proportion of such sudden deaths that result from a primary arrhythmia as opposed to thrombotic events such as MI, pulmonary embolism, or even stroke is unclear. Progressive HF represents another common cause of death. Results from three trials are presented in **40, 41**.

Although asymptomatic left ventricular systolic dysfunction has a better outlook compared to those with symptoms, the prognosis is related to LVEF (*Table 8*). The prognosis of diastolic heart failure is felt to be better than that resulting from systolic

---

Table 7 Factors associated with adverse prognosis in heart failure

Clinical features
◇ High NYHA class
◇ Third heart sound

Investigations
◇ Reduced peak oxygen consumption (VO_2 max)
◇ Reduced LVEF
◇ Increased pulmonary capillary wedge pressure
◇ Reduced cardiac index
◇ Hyponatraemia
◇ Anaemia
◇ Raised plasma noradrenaline (norepinephrine)
◇ Raised plasma BNP
◇ Decreased heart rate variability

BNP: brain natriuretic peptide; LVEF: left ventricular ejection fraction; NYHA: New York Heart Association; VO_2 max: maximum peak oxygen uptake.

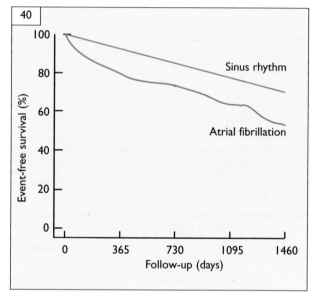

40 Results from the Studies of Left Ventricular Dysfunction (SOLVD) on atrial fibrillation and poorer outcomes in chronic heart failure.

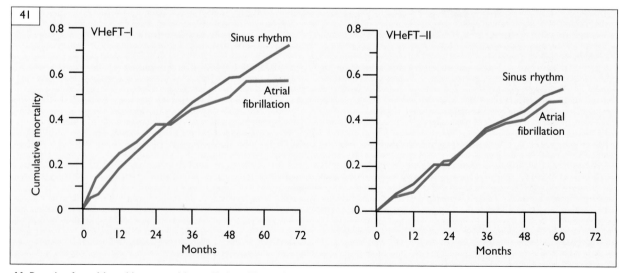

41 Results from Vasodilators in Heart Failure Trials (VHeFT)-I and -II on mortality and atrial fibrillation. (From Carson PE, *et al. Circulation* 1993;**87**(Suppl 6):1101.

dysfunction, with annual mortality ranging from 1.3–17.5% depending on the diagnostic definition used. Some authors have questioned whether the prognosis for patients with diastolic heart failure is actually as favourable as has been previously suggested, particularly in the elderly, and further data are necessary here.

The last decade has seen increasingly widespread use of drug therapies (e.g. angiotensin-converting enzyme (ACE) inhibitors and β-blockers) proven to enhance survival, improve symptoms, and delay progression of heart failure. Recent analysis of Framingham data has, encouragingly, revealed an upward trend in survival after the onset of HF in recent years, perhaps reflecting use of ACE inhibitors. Further improvements in mortality data are anticipated in response to increasing use of β-blockade. However, this trend notwithstanding, the mortality among Framingham patients diagnosed with HF in the 1990s still remained >50%.

The economic burden of chronic heart failure

Given the prevalence of this condition and the associated morbidity requiring frequent clinic visits and hospitalizations, HF is a costly condition to treat. Analyses reveal that HF accounts for between 1 and 2% of total health-care budgets. The bulk of HF-related spending is for hospitalization (*Table 9*), but investigations also account for a considerable proportion. Furthermore, the cost of long-term, evidence-based drug therapies, which aim to improve

survival, is a significant expense. Such therapies, however, also result in symptomatic improvement and, as a result, fewer hospital admissions, which will actually reduce overall expenditure. HF also results in indirect costs to countries. For example, younger patients may need to discontinue employment, and social support is frequently necessary, especially in older patients.

Although more widespread use of cost-effective treatments such as ACE inhibitors and β-blockers may reduce overall costs by reducing hospitalization, the projected increase in the prevalence of HF is likely to have the opposite effect. In addition, the use of modern, nonpharmacological therapies aimed at reducing mortality and morbidity is being evaluated. These interventions involve implantable cardioverter defibrillators (ICD) and dual chamber pacemakers, both of which represent potential acceleration in treatment costs. Thus, the economic burden of HF will continue to rise.

Summary

HF is a common medical condition with incidence rising due to an ageing population and improved survival following MI. It is associated with substantial morbidity and sufferers endure a poor quality of life, prior to a hastened death. The cost to health-care budgets is considerable, and likely to increase in the future. Therefore, preventative strategies need to be implemented urgently.

Table 8 Outcome of asymptomatic left ventricular dysfunction: impact (by relative risk) of each 5% reduction in left ventricular ejection fraction

Outcome	Relative risk	95% confidence intervals
Death	1.20	1.13–1.29
Hospitalization for heart failure	1.28	1.18–1.38
Onset of heart failure	1.20	1.13–1.26

Table 9 Impact of chronic heart failure on health-care expenditure

Country (year)	% of total health-care spending	% of costs due to hospitalization
New Zealand (1990)	1.4	67
France (1990)	1.9	64
UK (1990–1991)	1.2	60
The Netherlands (1994)	1.1	68
Sweden (1996)	2.0	74
USA (2000)	1.5	–
(From Berry C, *et al. Eur. J. Heart Failure* 2001;**3**:283.)		

Further reading

Berry C, Murdoch DR, McMurray JJ. Economics of chronic heart failure. *Eur. J. Heart Failure* 2001;3:283–291.

Davies MK, Hobbs FDR, Davis RC, *et al.* Prevalence of left ventricular systolic dysfunction and heart failure in the Echocardiographic Heart of England Screening Study; a population-based study. *Lancet* 2001;**358**:439–444.

Ho KK, Pinsky JL, Kannel WB, Levy D. The epidemiology of heart failure: the Framingham study. *J. Am. Coll. Cardiol.* 1993;**22**:6A–13A.

Kass DA, Bronzwaer JG, Paulus WJ. What mechanisms underlie diastolic dysfunction in heart failure? *Circ. Res.* 2004;**94**(12):1533–1542.

Levy D, Kenchaiah S, Larson MG, *et al.* Long-term trends in the incidence and survival with heart failure. *N. Engl. J. Med.* 2002;**347**:1397–1402.

McMurray JJ, Stewart S. Epidemiology, aetiology and prognosis of heart failure. *Heart* 2000;**83**:596–602.

Mendez GF, Cowie MR. The epidemiological features of heart failure in developing countries: a review of the literature. *Int. J. Cardiol.* 2001;**80**;213–219.

Sosin MD, Bhatia GS, Davis RC, Lip GY. Heart failure – the importance of ethnicity. *Eur. J. Heart Fail.* 2004;**6**(7):831–843.

Chapter two

Clinical features

Introduction

Since heart failure (HF) is a condition with high morbidity and mortality, and one for which treatments are available which can reduce mortality and improve quality of life, early recognition is important. It is important that general practitioners, physicians, and emergency department staff are familiar with the clinical features of HF to facilitate such early recognition, in order to allow early introduction of appropriate therapy. However, it is also important to be aware that the symptoms and signs of HF are nonspecific, and to have a low threshold for further investigation where there is any possibility of a diagnosis of HF. This chapter sets out the common clinical features and modes of presentation associated with HF, and discusses complications and prognosis of HF.

Mode of presentation

As HF represents the common final pathway of many cardiovascular disorders, presentation ranges from acute (for example following massive myocardial infarction [MI]) to insidious (for example in hypertensive heart disease). Figure **42** demonstrates the stages of progression seen in many patients with chronic HF. The clinical features listed below may occur in all patients with HF, but their relative importance may differ; using the above example, the patient with acute HF following MI may have gross signs of pulmonary oedema, but little or no peripheral signs of HF. The converse may well be true for the patient with hypertensive heart disease. The mode of presentation is likely to influence treatment strategy greatly initially, but once stabilized, chronic HF treatment will be similar for all patients.

42 Diagram to show the evolution of clinical stages of heart failure. HF: heart failure; LV: left ventricular.

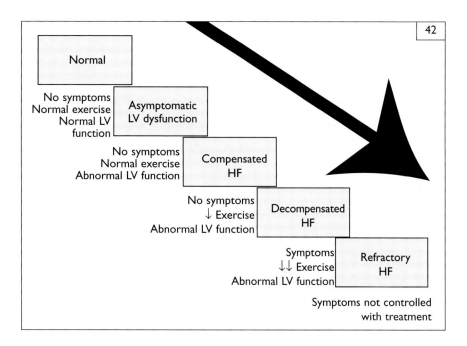

Symptoms of heart failure

GENERAL

HF has many causes, as described in Chapter 1. A high index of suspicion is necessary in patients with predisposing conditions, such as a previous history of MI, diabetes, or hypertension. It is important not to discount the diagnosis of HF in young patients, as dilated cardiomyopathy can occur at any age. If the diagnosis is not considered, such patients may be readily misdiagnosed as having asthma, for example.

Lethargy and general malaise

For many patients with chronic HF, the most debilitating symptom is tiredness. Patients may have difficulty sleeping due to other symptoms of HF, but lethargy is itself a feature of HF, and has a profound effect on patients' exercise capacity and quality of life, over and above that caused by breathlessness and other symptoms. Patients with HF also typically report increased muscle fatigue on exertion, contributing to reduced exercise capacity. Skeletal muscle metabolism has been shown to be abnormal in HF (*Table 10*). Some patients with HF may present only with feelings of general malaise, and careful questioning may be necessary to detect other symptoms of HF.

Loss of appetite

Patients with heart failure may complain of loss of appetite, which may be due to bowel oedema. Weight loss due to such anorexia may be masked by fluid accumulation, and become apparent only when diuretic therapy is instituted. Poor nutrition due to anorexia combined with reduced absorption from the oedematous bowel eventually results in cardiac cachexia, and the resulting reduction in muscle bulk compounds lethargy and breathlessness. Patients may also complain of right upper quadrant discomfort or pain, caused by liver congestion and capsular stretch.

Table 10 Muscle abnormalities in heart failure

✧ Wasting

✧ Impaired resting blood flow

✧ Limited capacity to enhance blood flow on exertion

✧ Increased fatigue

✧ Abnormal metabolism

✧ Early anaerobic metabolism

✧ Early intracellular acidosis

(From Harlan WR, *et al. Ann. Intern. Med.* 1977;**86**:133–138.)

BREATHLESSNESS

Shortness of breath is the most well known symptom of HF, but is a common symptom of many conditions, and therefore is not very specific for HF. Classically, patients complain of orthopnoea (breathlessness when lying flat), which may be quantified by asking how many pillows the patient uses in bed. Paroxysmal nocturnal dyspnoea (PND; episodic breathlessness waking the patient from sleep) is another classic symptom of HF and, again, the frequency of such episodes can be useful in quantifying severity. Not all patients complain of these symptoms, however, and their absence does not rule out the possibility of a diagnosis of HF.

Acute HF most often presents with extreme breathlessness of very sudden onset, such that the patient is often too breathless to talk. Diagnosis in this circumstance relies on clinical examination and investigation, although witnesses may be able to provide some clues. HF should always be considered in the acutely breathless patient. Where there is diagnostic doubt, a trial of a diuretic may result in rapid improvement in the patient with HF.

Patients with more insidious onset of HF may describe gradually worsening shortness of breath, and decreasing exercise tolerance over weeks or months. Cough may be an early symptom of HF, and some patients may complain of wheeze, caused by oedema of the bronchial tree, both of which may initially suggest the diagnosis of asthma.

PERIPHERAL OEDEMA

In some patients, the first symptom of HF may be development of peripheral oedema. The patient's usual posture determines the location of oedema: ambulant patients typically initially develop oedema of the ankles which resolves overnight; patients who are immobile may develop oedema predominantly over the sacrum. Oedema has many causes, particularly gravitational in immobile patients. Other causes of oedema may be mistaken for, or coexist with, HF (*Table 11*). Oedema is classically a sign of right-sided HF, for example in the patient with chronic obstructive pulmonary disease (cor pulmonale), but even in patients with predominant left-sided HF, oedema may be the main presenting feature with breathlessness less apparent.

Signs of heart failure

In some patients, clinical examination may make the diagnosis clear, but some patients with early HF may have few or no apparent clinical signs. In addition, the signs associated with HF have other

Table 11 Causes of oedema
◇ Heart failure
◇ Gravitational oedema
◇ Hypoproteinaemia
◇ Liver disease
◇ Nephrotic syndrome
◇ Lymphoedema
◇ Medications – calcium channel blockers, e.g. amlodipine

Table 12 Diagnostic sensitivity and specificity of clinical features of heart failure

Clinical features	Sensitivity (%)	Specificity (%)
Breathlessness	66	52
Orthopnea	21	81
PND	33	76
Oedema (history)	23	80
Tachycardia	7	99
Pulmonary crackles	13	91
Oedema (examination)	10	93
Third heart sound	31	95
Raised JVP	10	97

PND: paroxysmal nocturnal dyspnoea; JVP; jugular venous pulsation

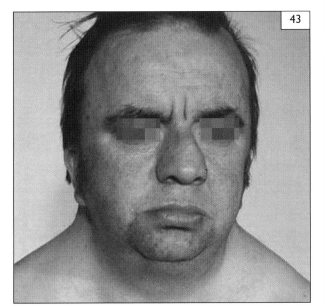

43 Noonan's syndrome – short webbed neck, low-set ears, high nasal bridge; may be subtle and present in adulthood.

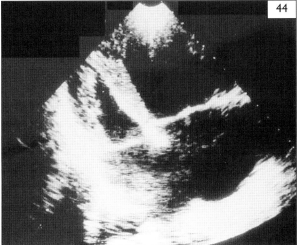

44 Atrial septal defect associated with Noonan's syndrome.

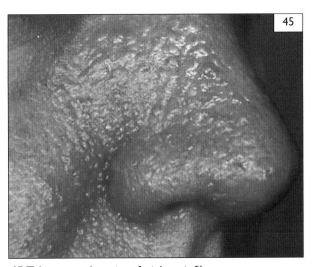

45 Tuberose sclerosis – facial angiofibroma.

causes which must be considered. *Table 12* presents the diagnostic sensitivity and specificity of clinical features of heart failure.

GENERAL EXAMINATION
Careful general examination may reveal useful information. Although HF is most commonly caused by ischaemic heart disease or hypertension, rarer causes must not be forgotten. Characteristic facies may be present. For example, Noonan's syndrome, which is associated with congenital heart disease (**43. 44**), or tuberose sclerosis (**45**) which may be associated with cardiac rhabdomyoma, which can be present as HF in

childhood. Systemic disorders such as gout (46, 47), dyslipidaemia (48), scleroderma (49, 50), connective tissue disorders (e.g. Ehlers–Danlos syndrome [51, 52] or Marfan syndrome [53], both associated with mitral valve prolapse), or neurofibromatosis (Von Recklinghausen syndrome [54–57, 76]) may provide clues. Hypothyroidism is associated with HF and the typical 'myxoedema facies' should not be missed (58–60).

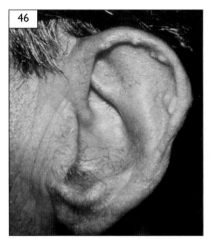

46 Chronic tophaceous gout.

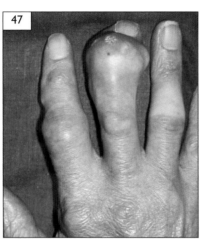

47 Chronic tophaceous gout.

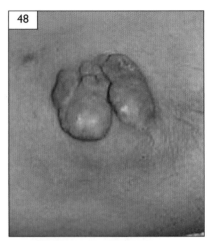

48 Cutaneous xanthomata in a patient with dyslipidaemia.

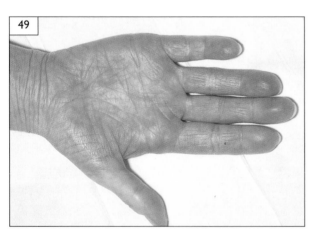

49 Scleroderma – tight, shiny skin over fingers, loss of finger pulp.

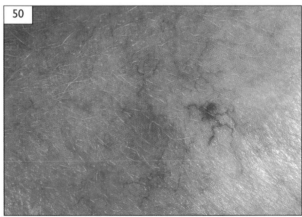

50 Skin in scleroderma showing telangiectasia.

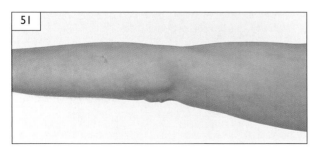

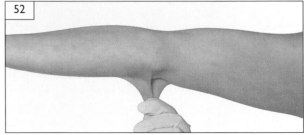

51, 52 Ehlers–Danlos syndrome – demonstration of skin laxity.

53 High arched palate in a patient with Marfan syndrome.

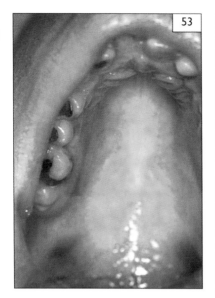

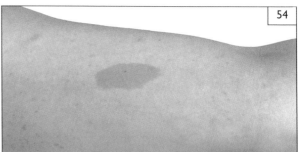

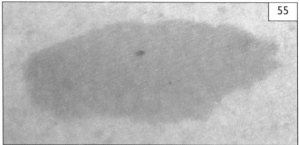

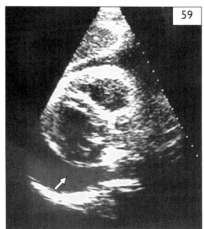

54–56 Von Recklinghausen syndrome – café-au-lait spots.

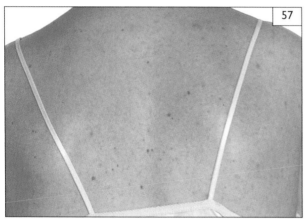

57 Von Recklinghausen's disease showing multiple neurofibromata.

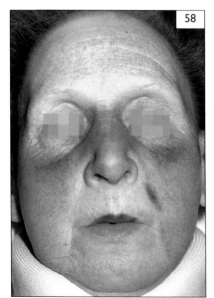

58 Myxoedema facies.

59 2D echocardiogram showing pericardial effusion due to hypothyroidism (arrow).

60 Electrical alternans in a patient with a large pericardial effusion. Alternating large and small QRS complexes caused by the heart swinging within the pericardial fluid.

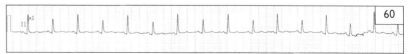

Carcinoid syndrome is associated with right-sided valvular abnormalities (**61–63**).

Patients with chronic HF are often anaemic (**64**). Anaemia may be due to poor nutrition, or alternatively due to anaemia of chronic disease. Anaemia may be sufficiently severe as to be apparent clinically. Recognition of anaemia is important, as correction may lead to an improvement in functional status.

Cachexia may occur in chronic HF (**65, 66**). Weight loss may be masked by accumulation of oedema, but loss of muscle bulk in the face and upper body may be clearly visible. Cachexia is a poor prognostic sign, and indicates severe HF.

Oedema may be the most obvious clinical sign of heart failure. It may range from subtle pitting to pressure over the tibia (**67, 68**), to gross oedema extending up to the abdomen and genitalia (**69**). Patients treated with diuretics may become dehydrated even in the presence of persistent oedema. Reduction of skin turgor and reduced urine output may accompany dehydration. During therapy, fluid status can be monitored by weighing.

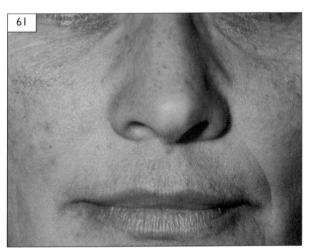

61 Facial telangiectasia in carcinoid syndrome.

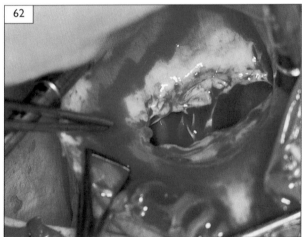

62 Fibrotic tricuspid valve in carcinoid syndrome.

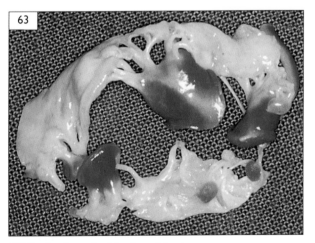

63 Excised carcinoid tricuspid valve.

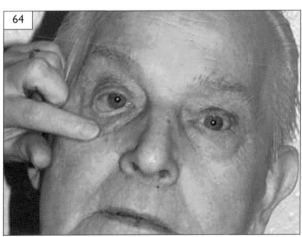

64 Patient with heart failure and clinical anaemia.

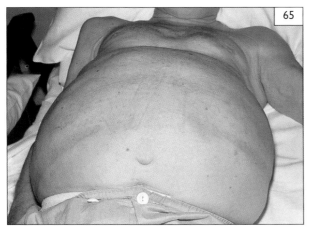

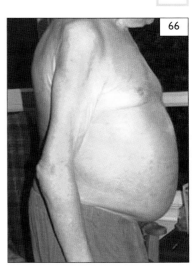

66 Cachexia – note severe loss of upper arm musculature.

65 Patient with advanced heart failure: note pitting oedema, ascites, and cachexia.

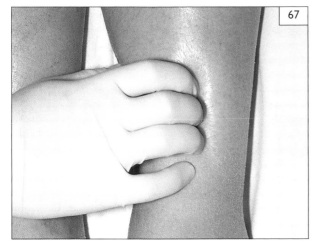

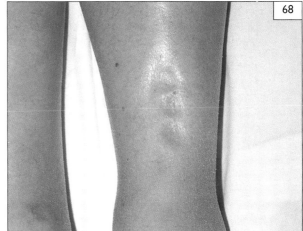

67, 68 Pitting peripheral oedema.

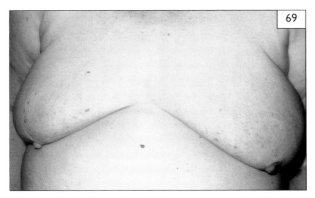

69 All body oedema.

Cardiovascular drugs, for example long-term therapy with amiodarone, may induce certain clinical features (70). Certain cardiac conditions may provide features on clinical examination, for example infective endocarditis (71–74).

CARDIOVASCULAR EXAMINATION

CARDIOVASCULAR EXAMINATION
Cardiovascular examination is obviously important in the detection of HF, and may provide additional information concerning the underlying cause. Full cardiovascular examination may be difficult in the

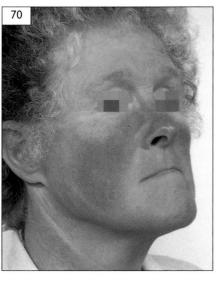

70 Amiodarone facial discoloration (slate-grey appearance).

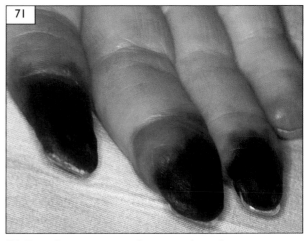

71 Digital gangrene in infective endocarditis.

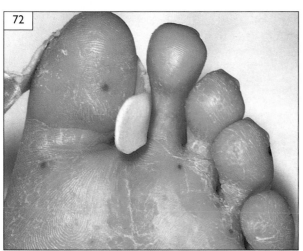

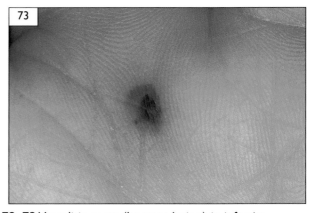

72, 73 Vasculitic spots (Janeway lesion) in infective endocarditis.

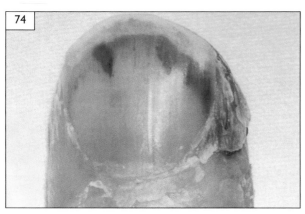

74 Splinter haemorrhages in infective endocarditis.

patient with acute breathlessness; in this situation a limited initial examination may be followed by detailed examination once therapy has commenced and symptoms have started to improve.

Pulse
Examination of the pulse often reveals tachycardia (compensating for reduced stroke volume), even in patients who are asymptomatic at rest. In acute HF, the radial pulse may be weak, and tachycardia may be extreme. Atrial fibrillation (AF) is common in HF, and the ventricular rate may be very rapid. Recognition and early treatment of AF may rapidly produce improvement in clinical status.

Jugular venous pulsation
The jugular venous pulsation (JVP) is regarded as a barometer of right atrial pressure, and may be raised in HF (75). It should be assessed with the patient lying at 45 degrees. It is useful to differentiate HF clinically from other causes of peripheral oedema (such as hypoproteinaemia, where the JVP is likely to be low), but it has low sensitivity for HF. It may not be visible in the obese patient, or the patient with acute HF and severe breathlessness. The absence of a raised JVP should not rule out the possibility of heart failure.

Palpation
Valve lesions may be associated with palpable thrills. A right ventricular heave may be present in patients with pulmonary hypertension and right-sided HF (for example, cor pulmonale). Palpation of the cardiac apex may show lateral displacement from the normal position (5th intercostal space, midclavicular line). The character of the apex beat may also be abnormal. A sustained, heaving apex may occur. All

75 Raised jugular venous pulsation.

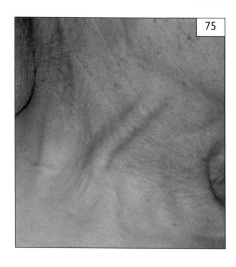

of these signs take time to develop, and may well be absent in patients with HF of acute onset.

Auscultation
Auscultation may be difficult in the breathless patient. Tachycardia may also mask signs. There may be a third or fourth heart sound (due to rapid ventricular filling or atrial contraction against a stiff left ventricle, respectively), or murmurs of underlying valve disease (or functional mitral regurgitation). The presence of a third heart sound is specific for HF, but has a high interobserver variability.

Blood pressure
Blood pressure measurement should be part of cardiovascular examination. High blood pressure should be detected, treated, and controlled. Rarely, unusual causes of hypertension, such as phaeochromocytoma (76, 77) and renal artery stenosis (78) should be considered as causes of HF.

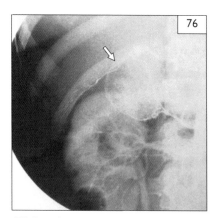

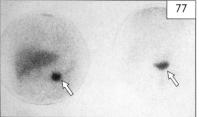

77 MIBG (meta-iodobenzyl guanidine) scan of phaeochromocytoma (arrows).

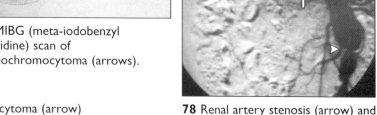

76 Renal angiogram showing phaeochromocytoma (arrow) (here associated with Von Recklinghausen syndrome).

78 Renal artery stenosis (arrow) and distal aortic stenosis (arrowhead).

RESPIRATORY EXAMINATION

Tachypnoea is a common finding, particularly in acute HF, where it may be accompanied by the use of accessory muscles of respiration. Cough may be apparent, and may be productive of pink, frothy sputum in acute pulmonary oedema. Percussion of the chest may demonstrate bilateral pleural effusions, which may not be equal in size. Auscultation often reveals fine end inspiratory crackles, which may be widespread in severe HF. However, crackles may also be caused by infection or pulmonary fibrosis, and it is also possible that wheeze may be the predominant finding in HF, due to oedema of the bronchial tree.

ABDOMINAL EXAMINATION

Ideally, examination of the abdomen should be carried out with the patient supine, but many patients with HF will not be able to tolerate this. Examination may reveal oedema of the abdominal wall or genitalia. Ascites is very often present (79), although commonly it is not clinically apparent, and tense ascites in the presence of oedema should prompt a search for other causes such as liver disease, although HF is still a possibility. Hepato-megaly due to congestion may be apparent. The liver edge will be smooth, is often tender, and may be pulsatile in the presence of tricuspid regurgitation.

Precipitating causes

In patients with documented HF, an episode of decompensation may be associated with infection, anaemia, ischaemia or infarction, or arrhythmia. Signs of these conditions may be apparent on clinical examination.

Objective confirmation

Although in patients with a suggestive history and multiple signs of HF the diagnosis may be made with some confidence, ideally all patients should have the diagnosis confirmed with objective evidence of cardiac dysfunction (see Chapter 4) as early as is practicable. A low threshold for investigation is necessary in those with equivocal history and clinical signs.

Classification

It is convenient to classify the severity of HF, using a simple scale such as the New York Heart Association (NYHA) system (Table 13). Increasing NYHA class is associated with decreased 1-year survival (although other factors such as echocardiographic parameters also help prognostic estimation), and provides an easy way to communicate disease severity with other health professionals. Patient progress may also be easily documented by noting change in their NYHA class.

Complications

THROMBOEMBOLISM

There is considerable evidence that thrombosis-related problems are more important in HF than was previously thought, and contribute significantly to the progression of the disease and mortality (80–82). Including stroke, thromboembolic complications may account for as much as 25% of noncardiac mortality in HF. Factors increasing the risk of thromboembolism in patients with HF include wall motion abnormalities or the presence of ventricular aneurysms (83, 84), immobility, AF, and low cardiac

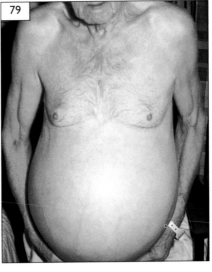

79 Ascites. (Photo courtesy of Dr SD Rosen.)

Table 13 New York Heart Association Classification		
Class I	Asymptomatic	No limitation of exercise capacity, but evidence of cardiac dysfunction on e.g. echocardiography.
Class II	Mild	Slight limitation of exercise capacity, with symptoms on significant exertion e.g. walking up several flights of stairs.
Class III	Moderate	Significant limitation of activities; symptoms on mild exertion but not at rest.
Class IV	Severe	Severely limited; symptoms at rest.

output. Stroke risk increases with decreasing left ventricular ejection fraction (LVEF): the Survival and Ventricular Enlargement (SAVE) study found a relative risk of 1.86 for patients with LVEF <28% compared to those with LVEF >35%.

AF is a known risk factor for thromboembolism, and it is accepted that most patients in AF with associated HF benefit from oral anticoagulation. The Stroke Prevention in Atrial Fibrillation (SPAF) trial found a relative risk of 1.9 for thromboembolism for patients with AF and HF compared to those with AF and no HF. Although AF may have accounted for many thromboembolic events seen in observational studies, patients with HF in sinus rhythm are also at increased thromboembolic risk.

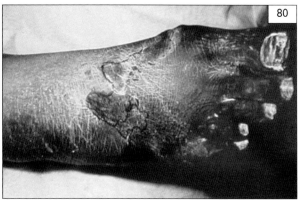

80 Peripheral emboli and gangrene due to a left ventricular thrombus.

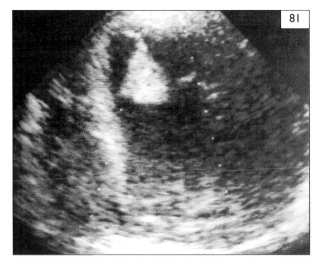

81 Apical left ventricular thrombus.

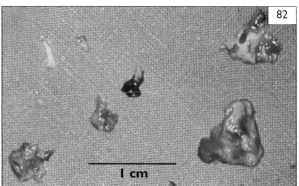

82 Hypertensive left ventricular dysfunction with peripheral emboli.

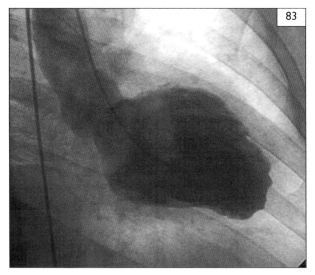

83 Apical left ventricular aneurysm, diastolic frame.

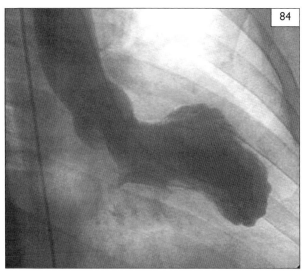

84 Apical left ventricular aneurysm, systolic frame.

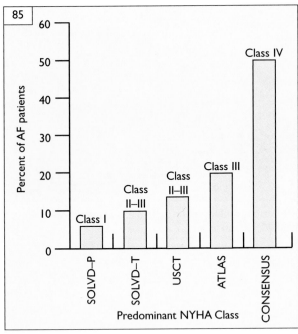

85 Prevalence of atrial fibrillation (AF) in landmark heart failure trials. NYHA: New York Heart Association. (For Trials see Appendix A.)

ARRHYTHMIA

Atrial fibrillation
As noted above, AF is common in HF. Estimates of prevalence range from 10 to 50% (**85**). AF may occur as a cause or as a result of HF, and the onset of AF in a patient with preexisting HF is a common cause of decompensation. Treatment of fast AF by cardioversion (where appropriate) or rate control may improve clinical status significantly. *Table 14* presents the risk factors for patients with atrial fibrillation at high risk of stroke and thromboembolism.

Ventricular arrhythmias
Many patients have frequent ventricular extrasystoles or runs of nonsustained ventricular tachycardia on 24-hour Holter monitoring (**86**). Malignant ventricular arrhythmias occur frequently in patients with severe HF. An episode of sustained ventricular tachycardia is associated with a high probability of recurrent arrhythmia and sudden death. Patients with hypokalaemia (aggravated by diuretic therapy), hypomagnesaemia, recurrent ischaemia, or infarction are at particularly high risk of malignant ventricular arrythmia. In addition, antiarrhythmic drugs including digoxin, as well as other drugs (such as tricyclic antidepressants and certain antihistamines) may predispose to arrhythmias. Increasing use of implantable cardioverter defibrillators (ICD) may lead to increasing survival in patients at risk of ventricular arrhythmias.

Table 14 Identifying the patient with atrial fibrillation at high risk of stroke and thromboembolism

Clinical and echocardiographic factors	Relative risk (95% confidence interval)	P value
Age (per decade)	1.5 (1.1–2.0)	0.006
Hypertension	1.5 (0.9–2.5)	0.13
Stroke or TIA	3.5 (1.8–6.7)	<0.001
Diabetes	1.7 (1.0–2.9)	0.05
Heart failure	1.4 (0.8–2.3)	0.16
LV dysfunction*	2.5 (1.5–4.4)	<0.001

n=1010; 847 >65 years or with ≥1 clinical risk factor or moderate/poor LV function. * Moderate to severe LV systolic dysfunction via 2D echo. NB. Left atrial diameter by M-mode echo did not predict stroke (relative risk, 1.02/mm; P=0.10). LV: left ventricular; TIA: transient ischaemic attack. (From Atrial Fibrillation Investigators. *Arch. Intern. Med.* 1998;**158**:1316–1320.)

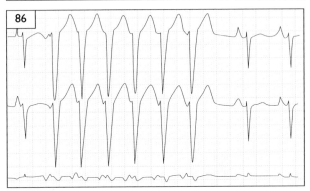

86 Section of a 24-hour Holter monitor electrocardiographic reading, showing a run of nonsustained ventricular tachycardia.

Further reading
Coats AJS. What causes the symptoms of heart failure? *Heart* 2001;**86**:574–578.
Fonseca C, Morais H, Mota T, Matias F, Costa C, Gouveia–Oliveira A, Ceia F; EPICA Investigators. The diagnosis of heart failure in primary care: value of symptoms and signs. *Eur. J. Heart Fail.* 2004;**6**(6):795–800, 821–822.
Loh E, Sutton MS, Wun CC, *et al*. Ventricular dysfunction and the risk of stroke after myocardial infarction. *N. Engl. J. Med.* 1997;**336**:251–257 (SAVE study).
SOLVD investigators. Effect of enalapril on mortality and the development of heart failure in asymptomatic patients with reduced left ventricular ejection fractions. *N. Engl. J. Med.* 1992;**327**:685–691.
SPAF investigators. Predictors of thromboembolism in atrial fibrillation I. Clinical features of patients at risk. The Stroke Prevention in Atrial Fibrillation Investigators. *Ann. Intern. Med.* 1992;**116**:1–5.

Chapter three

Pathogenesis

Determinants of ventricular function

Ventricular function can be divided into two separate stages, contraction (systole) and relaxation (diastole). Each of these opposite functions is dependent upon a multitude of factors both intrinsic and extrinsic to the heart. Systolic ventricular function can be quantified by measurement of the cardiac output (CO), usually around 5 l/minute. CO is a function of heart rate and stroke volume. These parameters, in turn, are dependent upon certain physiological indices (87), and vary according to the body's need.

Cardiac output is dependent largely on loading conditions immediately preceding and during systole. Left ventricular preload is determined by the volume of blood occupying the ventricle at the initiation of contraction (end-diastolic volume, EDV), whereas afterload is the resistance to ejection, the systemic vascular resistance (SVR). Stroke volume (typically 70 ml at rest) is greatly influenced by myocardial contractility but is also dependent on valvular competence and synchronous contraction of the entire ventricle.

Furthermore, the autonomic nervous system has a major influence upon heart rate and stroke volume. For example, parasympathetic stimulation decreases the heart rate (negatively chronotropic), whereas sympathetic stimulation has the opposite effect (positively chronotropic) and increases contractility (positively inotropic) and vascular resistance. Adequate relaxation of the ventricle is necessary for filling before the next contraction, and is dependent upon heart rate and ventricular compliance, which may be adversely affected by hypertrophy or fibrosis.

It is therefore clear that normal ventricular function is dependent upon a fine balance between multiple factors, and that any abnormality of these factors could contribute to the development of heart failure (HF).

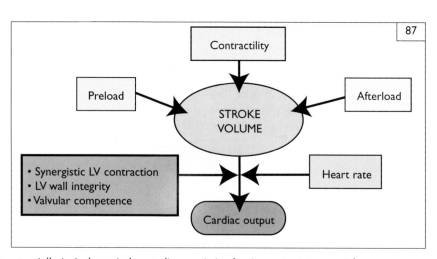

87 Determinants of left ventricular function. Cardiac function depends upon the interaction of four factors that regulate the volume of blood expelled by the heart (cardiac output, CO): contractility, preload, afterload, and heart rate. The first three determine the volume of blood expelled with each beat (stroke or ejection volume), while the heart rate affects the CO by varying the number of contractions per unit time. These four intrinsic regulators of heart function are all influenced by the nervous system. In the failing heart, especially in ischaemic heart disease, it is also important to consider some purely mechanical factors, such as the synergy of ventricular contraction, the integrity of the septum, and the competence of the atrioventricular valves. LV: left ventricular.

Pathogenesis

The clinical syndrome of HF results from the complex interplay of a number of physiological systems. Myocardial insults (e.g. from infarction or chronic hypertension) lead to a variety of adaptive changes, which may temporarily stabilize any resulting deterioration in myocardial performance.

However, with increasing severity of insult, or with increasing demand, these initially adaptive responses undermine overall cardiac performance and are, therefore, ultimately maladaptive.

The mechanisms which eventuate cardiac failure will be discussed in this chapter, with reference to current and potential treatment strategies.

Frank–Starling law

According to the Frank–Starling law, increasing muscle length results in increasing contractile power up to a threshold, after which further increases in length lead to functional deterioration. In normal ventricles, there exists a positive association between cardiac filling and cardiac output (88). The onset of mild ventricular dysfunction causes the ventricle to respond by increasing preload in order to achieve the same level of performance (points B–C). Thus, the failing heart compensates by increasing left ventricular end-diastolic pressure (LVEDP), and the normal curve is right-shifted with the steepness diminished. With worsening function, however, progressive increases in LVEDP lead to pulmonary congestion and exertional dyspnoea. Further deterioration is associated with an inability to normalize resting CO, and is characterized by severe HF.

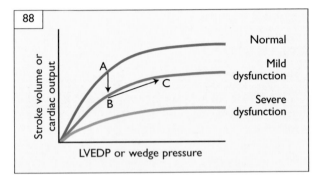

88 Idealized Frank–Starling curves produced by worsening ventricular function in heart failure. In ventricles with normal cardiac performance there is a steep and positive relationship between increased cardiac filling pressures (as estimated from the left ventricular end-diastolic pressure [LVEDP] or pulmonary capillary wedge pressure) and increased stroke volume or cardiac output (top curve). During progression from mild to severe myocardial dysfunction, the relationship shifts to the right (i.e. a higher filling pressure is required to achieve the same cardiac output) and is flattened, so that continued increases in left heart filling pressures lead to minimal increases in cardiac output, at the possible expense of pulmonary oedema. The onset of mild heart failure results in an initial reduction in cardiac function (point B), a change that can be normalized, at least at rest, by raising the LVEDP via fluid retention (point C). In comparison, normalization of stroke volume is not attainable in severe dysfunction (bottom curve).

Neurohormonal mechanisms

Activation of several neurohormonal mechanisms is central to the development of HF, and appreciation of these pathways has enabled the development of important pharmacological therapies. The consequences of certain neurohormonal responses may be apparent in the clinical signs of HF. The mechanisms highlighted in *Table 15* will be focused upon in this section, and the ensuing modifications are illustrated in **89**.

Table 15 Neurohormonal mechanisms involved in the pathogenesis of heart failure

Sympathetic nervous system ✧ Tachycardia ✧ Increased contractility ✧ Vasoconstriction and increased peripheral vascular resistance ✧ Activation of RAAS ✧ Reduced HRV	Natriuretic peptides ✧ Increased sodium excretion
	Vasopressin ✧ Increased water retention
	Endothelins
	Nitric oxide
RAAS ✧ Sodium and water retention ✧ Vasoconstriction ✧ Increased sympathetic activity ✧ Interstitial fibrosis	Inflammatory cytokines, e.g. TNFα
	HRV: heart rate variability; RAAS: renin–angiotensin–aldosterone system; TNFα: tumour necrosis factor alpha.

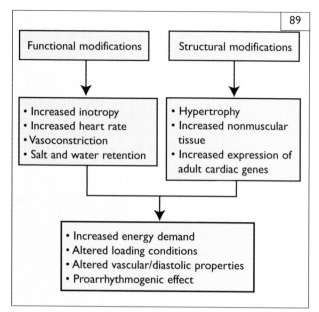

89 Functional and structural modifications following neurohormonal stimulation in heart failure.

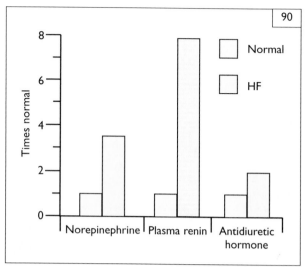

90 Hormones in heart failure. Plasma levels of norepinephrine, renin activity, and antidiuretic hormone are increased two- to eightfold when compared with normal subjects, in patients with stable chronic heart failure (HF) treated with digitalis but not diuretics or vasodilators. (From Francis GS, *et al. Ann. Intern. Med.* 1984;**101**:370.)

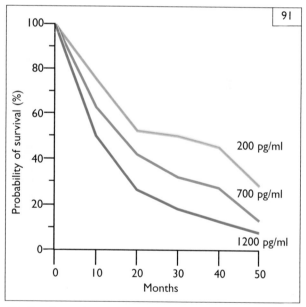

91 Graph to show the probability of survival in patients with advanced heart failure according to plasma norepinephrine concentration. Survival was inversely related to the degree of norepinephrine activation, a presumed reflection of worsening cardiac function. The time to 50% survival was approximately 30 months in patients with normal norepinephrine levels (200 pg/ml), but was only 10 months in those with marked hypersecretion (1200 pg/ml). (From Cohn JN, *et al. N. Engl. J. Med.* 1984;**311**:819.)

SYMPATHETIC NERVOUS SYSTEM

Left ventricular systolic dysfunction is characterized by dominance of the sympathetic nervous system. Sympathetic stimulation results in increased heart rate and myocardial contractility, both of which increase energy utilization. Heart rate variability (an index of autonomic function) is reduced in response to sympathetic dominance, and this reduction is associated with a higher risk of sudden death. Furthermore, sympathetically-mediated peripheral vasoconstriction leads to an increase in SVR, with subsequent rise in ventricular wall stress predisposing to myocardial hypertrophy. The renal vascular resistance is similarly increased, and the renin–angiotensin–aldosterone system (see also below), already activated by a reduction in renal perfusion, is further triggered by adrenergic release of renin. Direct effects of sympathetic overactivity on the myocardium include induction of myocyte apoptosis.

These changes represent adaptive phenomena, which maintain CO in the short term. With time, however, these responses become blunted, perhaps due to down-regulation of post-synaptic β receptors and depletion of norepinephrine at nerve endings. Clearly, sympathetic stimulation is manifested clinically in, for example, tachycardia or cool, cyanosed peripheries. Sympathetic overactivity is also reflected in high circulating levels of catecholamines (90). Indeed, plasma norepinephrine concentrations have been shown to be inversely associated with survival (91).

Recent studies have shown significant mortality benefit resulting from the use of β-blocker drugs in chronic, stable HF (covered further in Chapter 6), including reductions in sudden death. Furthermore, studies have also reported significant symptomatic improvement.

RENIN–ANGIOTENSIN–ALDOSTERONE SYSTEM

Although myocardial dysfunction is usually the primary cause of HF, the kidneys, which receive 25% of the CO, play a vital part in its pathophysiology. Inappropriate stimulation of the renin–angiotensin–aldosterone system (RAAS), conferring a state of hyperaldosteronism, drives the retention of sodium and water, leading to expansion of intravascular and extravascular volumes and the development of congestive HF. The development of drugs that interfere with this axis has been fundamental in the recent management of patients with HF. The RAAS is illustrated in 92.

Stimulation of the RAAS is an important physiological mechanism that is called upon in times of stress resulting from vascular depletion (e.g.

prolonged vomiting). The proteolytic enzyme, renin, is released by the juxtaglomerular apparatus within the kidney in response to diminished renal perfusion and sodium delivery that occur with dehydration. Cardiac dysfunction causes diminished renal perfusion despite retention of the circulating volume, and this activates renin production. Furthermore, β-adrenergic stimulation also promotes renin release. Renin acts upon angiotensinogen, a 14-amino acid peptide synthesized by the liver, forming angiotensin I. This decapeptide is cleaved of two amino acids by angiotensin-converting enzyme (ACE, abundant in the lungs and vasculature), to form the active molecule, angiotensin II. Angiotensin II induces intense systemic and renal efferent vasoconstriction (via sympathetic stimulation), stimulates thirst, and promotes sodium and water reabsorption in the proximal nephron. In addition, angiotensin II acts upon the zona glomerulosa of the adrenal cortex (as well as vascular endothelial and smooth muscle cells) to produce the mineralocorticoid aldosterone. This steroid stimulates sodium and water reabsorption in the distal collecting duct in the kidney. Thus, the overall effect of RAAS activation is fluid retention and vasoconstriction. Aldosterone has also been shown to effect ventricular remodelling (see below), a process causing further cardiac dysfunction; this involves initiation of synthesis of collagens by fibroblasts. Aldosterone may also adversely affect baroreceptor function and heart rate variability.

Hence, the activation of the RAAS is a maladaptive response to cardiac dysfunction. Circulating levels of renin (90), angiotensin II, and aldosterone are elevated in patients with congestive HF. Pharmacological targets within this axis are readily apparent, and the benefits of ACE inhibition in the management of systolic dysfunction are clear. More recently, angiotensin II receptor blockers have been shown to be of value in HF, and aldosterone antagonists have been associated with significant survival and symptomatic benefit (see also Chapter 5).

NATRIURETIC PEPTIDE FAMILY

Natriuretic peptides have recently attracted much attention as useful tools in the diagnosis and prognostication of cardiac diseases. There are three members of this family: atrial natriuretic peptide (ANP), brain natriuretic peptide (BNP) and C-type natriuretic peptide (CNP). ANP consists of 28 amino acids, and is made in, and released by, atrial tissue in response to myocyte stretch. BNP is synthesized predominantly by ventricular myocardium, and is released as a 108-amino acid precursor, Pro-BNP; the

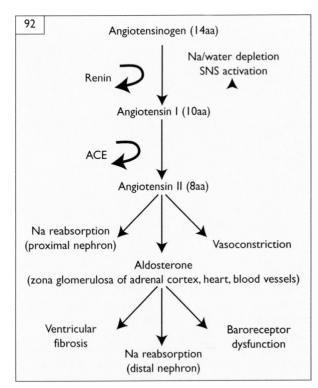

92 Activation of the renin–angiotensin–aldosterone system. aa: amino acid; ACE: angiotensin-converting enzyme; Na: sodium; SNS: sympathetic nervous system.

active hormone is a 32-amino acid peptide. Pro-BNP is cleaved to form BNP and an inactive, 76-amino acid peptide, N-terminal Pro-BNP, which has a longer half-life than BNP. CNP is principally expressed in the central nervous system.

There are three natriuretic peptide receptors, NPR-A, -B and -C. The physiological effects are mediated by receptors A and B, via the cyclic guanosine monophosphate (cGMP) second messenger system. Clearance of both ANP and BNP is dependent upon binding to NPR-C, and degradation by the enzyme neutral endopeptidase.

Unlike activation of the RAAS, ANP and BNP have a number of advantageous effects in the setting of cardiac dysfunction (93). As their names suggest, they induce loss of sodium and water by inhibiting renal sodium reabsorption. In addition, natriuretic peptides appear to attenuate sympathetic drive and reduce vascular tone. Interestingly, these peptides may actually have a favourable impact upon the RAAS.

Plasma levels of BNP are higher in patients with HF compared to normal subjects, with levels rising with worsening class. Furthermore, higher concentrations have independently predicted adverse prognosis in those with HF, illustrated in **94**. Higher values also appear to be associated with sudden cardiac death in patients with HF.

93 Representation of the effects of elevated plasma natriuretic peptides in chronic heart failure. Atrial natriuretic peptide (ANP) and brain natriuretic peptide (BNP) may increase (+) the rate of sodium excretion and reduce (−) the effects of the renin–angiotensin and sympathetic nervous systems and endothelin (ET-1); the net effect of these actions is reduced preload and afterload. A similar elevation in inducible nitric oxide synthase (iNOS) is seen in humans with severe heart failure. These initially homeostatic mechanisms paradoxically contribute to the pathophysiology of the failing myocardium. (Adapted from Baig M, et al. Am. Heart J. 1998;**135**:S217.)

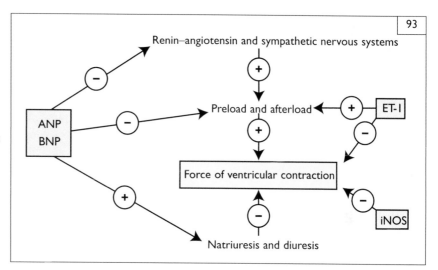

94 Graph to show the relationship between survival and brain natriuretic peptide (BNP). Kaplan–Meier survival curves in patients with chronic heart failure show that survival is significantly lower in patients with BNP >73 pg/ml compared with those with BNP <73 pg/ml (p <0.0001). (From Tsutamoto T, et al. *Circulation* 1997;**96**:509.)

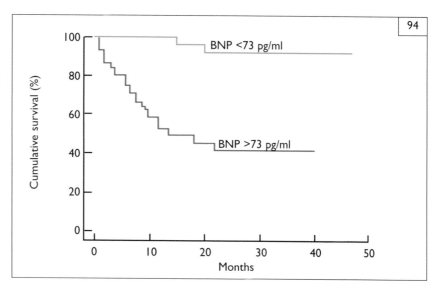

Pharmacological manipulation of these peptides has focused on two approaches. Firstly, recombinant BNP (nesiritide) has shown some promise in early trials of treatment of decompensated HF, although further data are required before achieving widespread use. Secondly, vasopeptidase inhibitors (e.g. omapatrilat), which inhibit both ACE and neutral endopeptidase (NEP) (which degrades the natriuretic peptides) have been developed. However, trial results have been rather disappointing so far.

VASOPRESSIN

Vasopressin, also known as antidiuretic hormone (ADH), is a peptide hormone released by the posterior pituitary gland. In health, it plays an important role in the maintenance of plasma osmolality, and acts by increasing the permeability of water in the collecting ducts of nephrons. Plasma vasopressin levels are elevated in patients with left ventricular systolic dysfunction, irrespective of the presence of symptoms (90). Such increased levels persist despite the reduction in plasma osmolality apparent in many patients with HF, and may contribute to the development of hyponatraemia. Indeed, hyponatraemia is associated with an adverse prognosis in HF (95), perhaps, in part, reflecting high circulating vasopressin levels.

ENDOTHELINS AND NITRIC OXIDE

Endothelin (ET) is an endothelium-derived peptide (21 amino acids) which has three subtypes, ET-1, -2, and -3. All three subtypes cause intense peripheral vasoconstriction by acting upon arterial smooth muscle cells via ET type A receptors. Indeed, ET-1 is ten times more potent a vasoconstrictor than angiotensin II. ET-A stimulation may also induce myocyte hypertrophy. Stimulation of type B receptors has been associated with aldosterone release. ET-1 levels have been shown to be elevated in the plasma of patients with HF; levels are associated with the severity of HF and, of note, with high pulmonary vascular resistance.

ET antagonists (e.g. bosentan, a specific ET-1 antagonist) have been studied in patients with pulmonary hypertension and HF. While bosentan appears to be effective in the management of patients with primary pulmonary hypertension, trials in patients with chronic HF have not suggested benefit over placebo so far. Studies involving tezosentan, a dual ET antagonist, show that these agents may be of benefit in acute HF.

Nitric oxide (NO) appears to have an important role in a number of conditions, including cardiovascular and neurological diseases. It is synthesized by the enzyme nitric oxide synthase (NOS), from the amino acid precursor, L-arginine. There are two isoforms of NOS (NOS-2 and NOS-3) that are prevalent within myocardium. Nitric oxide is recognized as having favourable, vasodilatory effect upon the vascular endothelium, which may be advantageous in HF by reducing vascular resistance. However, whether it is as directly beneficial to the myocardium is less clear. NOS-2 is an inducible enzyme, whose activity may

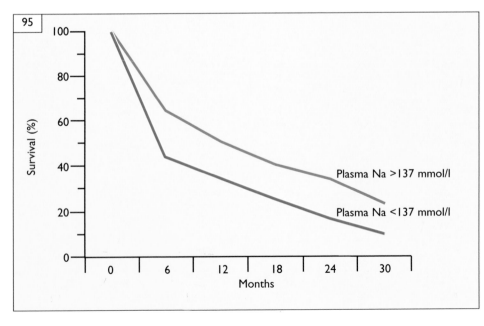

95 Graph to show the relationship between survival and plasma sodium levels in severe heart failure. Survival of patients with normal plasma sodium concentration (blue line) was significantly higher than survival of patients with hyponatraemia (red line). (From Lee WH, et al. *Circulation* 1986;**73**:257.)

be upregulated in response to certain stimuli including inflammatory cytokines such as tumour necrosis factor-alpha (TNF-α), and whose activity is increased in the failing heart. Thus, NO may mediate the negatively inotropic effects of TNF-α. Furthermore, NO may itself impair cellular energy production, stimulate production of damaging reactive oxygen species, and influence remodelling by inducing apoptosis (see below).

TUMOUR NECROSIS FACTOR-α

TNF-α is a 157-amino acid proinflammatory cytokine whose synthesis is increased in response to various infectious or inflammatory stimuli. TNF-α interacts with two distinct receptors: TNFR-1, which is soluble, and TNFR-2. TNF-α contributes to inflammatory cascades by inducing chemotaxis of phagocytic leucocytes, and promoting leucocyte adhesion to sites of inflammation. Clinical effects include initiation of fever, hypotension, and cachexia.

Interest in TNF-α and HF has grown since the discovery of increased circulating levels in patients with severe HF, especially in those with cachexia. Cardiac expression of TNF-α in end-stage HF is greatly increased compared to that of normal hearts, possibly resulting from increased production by failing myocardial tissue. Animal studies have shown that TNF-α itself exerts a negatively inotropic effect on myocardium; other effects may include induction of (cultured) myocyte hypertrophy, uncoupling of β-adrenoceptors, and metalloproteinase activation.

Large scale trials of TNF-α binding agents (soluble receptor proteins and antibodies) in HF have been conducted, but were terminated early without having demonstrated clinical benefit.

Ventricular remodelling

The myocardium undergoes certain changes in response to various pathological conditions in order to attempt to maintain performance. For example, in response to myocardial infarction (MI), after expansion of the infarct zone remote areas of ventricular myocardium may become hypertrophied. Similarly, following pressure overload (e.g. due to chronic hypertension or aortic stenosis) or volume overload (due to mitral valve incompetence), the left ventricle characteristically responds by developing concentric hypertrophy and dilatation, respectively. These are examples of the end-results of remodelling, and although cardiac performance in the face of these insults may be temporarily improved, continued damage precipitates further adverse remodelling, ultimately leading to HF.

Several ultrastructural processes contribute to ventricular remodelling, and their roles will be discussed in this section.

ALTERATIONS IN MYOCYTE STRUCTURE AND FUNCTION

Various stimuli (e.g. wall stress and TNF-α) influence cardiac myocytes to experience changes in morphological shape (e.g. become elongated) or to undergo hyperplasia, with the net effect being myocardial hypertrophy and increased myocardial mass. In addition, growth factors may also effect alterations in the ratio of fetal to adult gene expression, which may, in turn, alter myocyte function.

The contractile performance of individual myocytes may also be impaired, as suggested by various experimental observations, although whether these observed alterations are causes or effects of HF is unclear. Examples of reported changes that might adversely affect contractility include altered handling of ionized calcium, altered expression of the actual contractile proteins, and diminished myocyte energy reserves.

Ultimately, remodelling is associated with myocyte loss. This may occur by necrotic or apoptotic mechanisms. Myocyte necrosis may, of course, result from MI, which can initiate remodelling, but may also be a feature of ventricular hypertrophy where diminished subendocardial perfusion has been observed. Alternatively, apoptosis, an encoded cell death, has been observed in histological studies of failing myocardium. Possible apoptotic stimuli include angiotensin II, β-adrenergic stimulation, and NO.

ALTERATIONS IN THE EXTRACELLULAR MATRIX

Structural modifications in the failing heart include chamber dilatation and the accumulation of fibrous tissue. The myocardium consists of myocytes supported by an extracellular matrix (ECM) composed of collagens (principally types I and III), which are produced by fibroblasts. In the late 1980s, it was demonstrated that the ECM of failing myocardium undergoes alterations in composition. For example, type III collagen was more prevalent than type I in tissue obtained from subjects with idiopathic dilated cardiomyopathy.

ECM maintenance is a function of the interplay between two groups of enzymes, the matrix metalloproteinases (MMPs), which increase collagen breakdown, and their tissue inhibitors (TIMPs), which counteract this degradation. Thus, regulation of the ECM is a dynamic process; relative MMP dominance results in myocyte slippage and chamber dilatation, whereas TIMP dominance promotes fibrosis and reduced chamber compliance, which manifests as diastolic dysfunction. Synthesis of these enzymes appears to be modulated by various growth factors and inflammatory cytokines, including TNF-α.

Studies of failing human hearts have revealed increased MMP production and diminished TIMP expression, and much interest has focused on the potential therapeutic benefits of MMP inhibitors.

Summary

An intricate network of pathophysiological changes eventually leads to the clinical spectrum of features observed in patients with cardiac dysfunction. Many of these alterations are initially adaptations to preserve function, with ultimately deleterious and self-perpetuating effects. Further understanding will promote development of newer approaches to treatment.

Further reading

Bristow MR. Why does the myocardium fail? Insights from basic science. *Lancet* 1998;**352** (Suppl. I):8–14.

De Lemos JA, McGuire DK, Drazner MH. B-type natriuretic peptide in cardiovascular disease. *Lancet* 2003;**362**(9380):316–322.

Janicki JS, Brower GL, Gardner JD, Chancey AL, Stewart JA Jr. The dynamic interaction between matrix metalloproteinase activity and adverse myocardial remodelling. *Heart Fail. Rev.* 2004;**9**(10):33–42.

Kalantar–Zadeh K, Block G, Horwich T, Fonarow GC. Reverse epidemiology of conventional cardiovascular risk factors in patients with chronic heart failure. *J. Am. Coll. Cardiol.* 2004;**43**(8):1439–1444.

Weber KT. Aldosterone in congestive heart failure. *N. Engl. J. Med.* 2001;**345**:1689–1697.

Chapter four

Investigations

Introduction

Patients with heart failure (HF) often present with nonspecific symptoms and signs (Chapter 2). In addition, the diagnosis of HF should always be supported by objective evidence of cardiac dysfunction (typically echocardiographic). Therefore, a low threshold is needed for investigation of patients with suspected HF. Knowledge of investigations used in HF and ability to interpret their results are important for all physicians and emergency department staff.

The recent UK National Institute for Clinical Excellence (NICE) guidelines recommend the algorithm shown in **96** for the diagnosis of HF.

96 Algorithm summarizing recommendations from the UK National Institute for Clinical Excellence for the diagnosis of heart failure. BNP: brain natriuretic peptide; ECG: electrocardiography; FBC: full blood count; LFT: liver function test; NTproBNP: N terminal pro-brain natriuretic peptide; TFT: thyroid function test; U&E: urine and electrolytes.

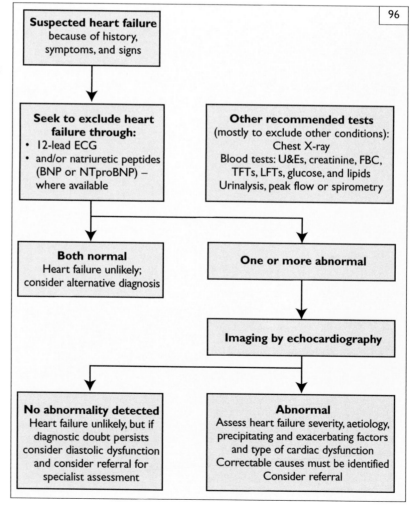

Electrocardiogram

The electrocardiogram (ECG) is a simple, non-invasive tool. All patients with suspected HF should have an ECG, and patients with acute severe HF require serial ECGs to exclude myocardial infarction (MI) as an underlying cause. A completely normal ECG has a high negative predictive value for HF, although further confirmatory investigations (such as echocardiography) are still recommended if there is any doubt.

The ECG in patients with HF may show abnormalities of rate, rhythm, conduction, and cardiac size. Tachycardia is almost universal in patients not taking rate-limiting medication (such as β-blockers). Atrial fibrillation (AF) is also frequently seen, and may be rapid (97) but occasionally be slow (98) or be related to preexcitation (99, 100). The latter may also lead to other tachyarrhythmias. Frequent ectopic beats are also common in the resting ECG of patients with HF (101, 102).

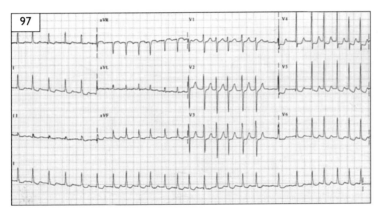

97 Electrocardiogram showing fast atrial fibrillation; note the irregular rhythm and absence of p waves.

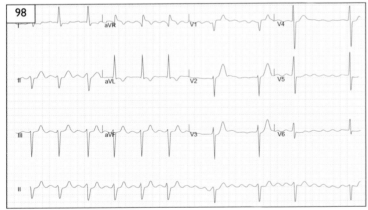

98 Electrocardiogram showing slow atrial fibrillation/atrial flutter.

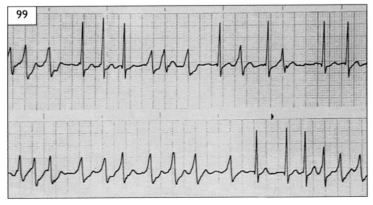

99 Electrocardiogram showing atrial fibrillation and preexcitation.

100 Electrocardiogram showing atrial fibrillation and preexcitation, proceeding to a very rapid ventricular response equivalent to ventricular flutter.

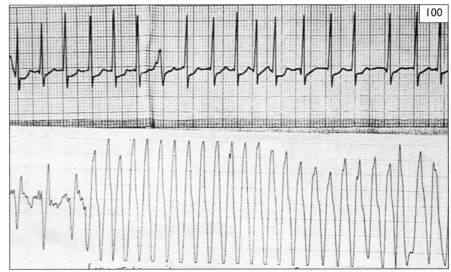

101 Electrocardiogram showing ventricular bigeminy. Each sinus QRS complex is followed by a ventricular extrasystole.

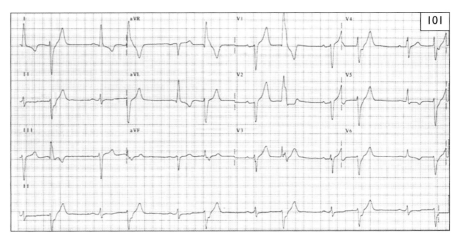

102 Electrocardiogram showing ventricular extrasystole, triplets, and couplets.

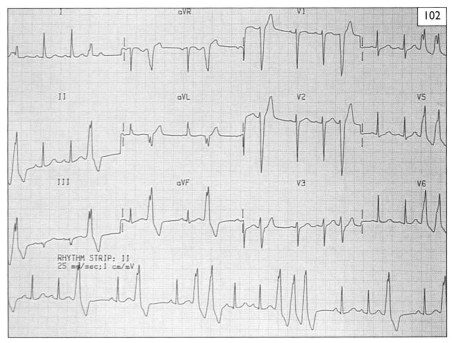

Conduction abnormalities such as heart block may provoke or exacerbate HF (103–105). However, such arrhythmias are not always apparent on a single ECG and a 24-hour Holter monitor may reveal conduction abnormalities and sinus node disease (106–110).

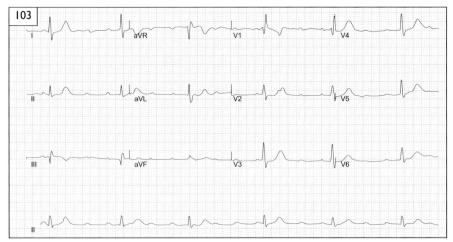

103 Electrocardiogram showing complete heart block.

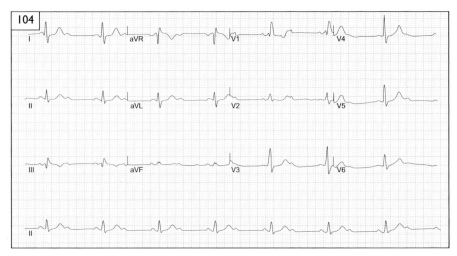

104 Electrocardiogram showing 2:1 atrioventricular block.

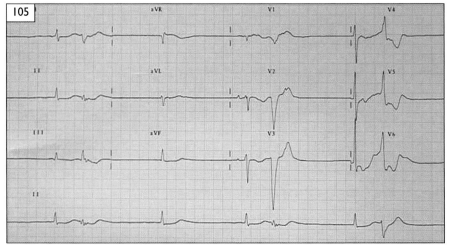

105 Electrocardiogram showing sinus rhythm degenerating to nodal bradycardia with ventricular ectopics.

106 Electrocardiogram showing sinus arrest, sinoatrial block with multiple pauses up to 14 seconds.

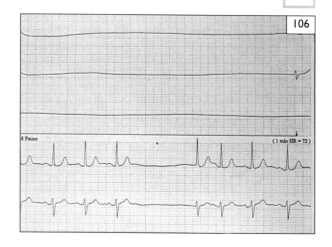

107 Segment of 24-hour Holter electrocardiogram showing sinus arrest with multiple pauses.

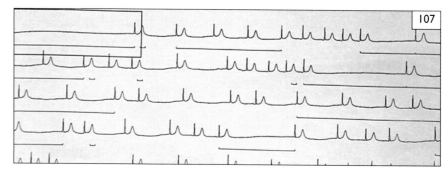

108 Segment of 24-hour Holter electrocardiogram showing a 14 second pause.

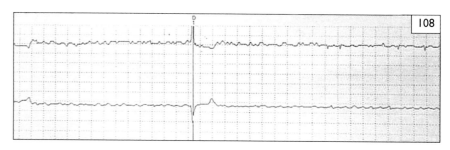

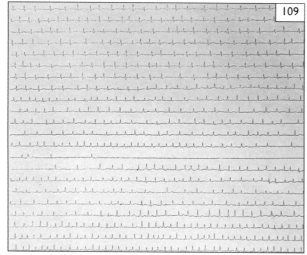

109 Segment of 24-hour Holter electrocardiogram showing sinus arrest.

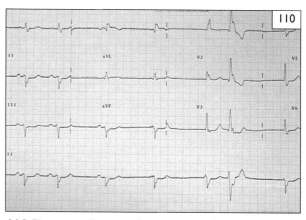

110 Electrocardiogram showing sinus rhythm degenerating to nodal bradycardia. (Left axis deviation, right bundle branch block, P mitrale, and a ventricular extrasystole.)

The ECG may provide information concerning the underlying cause of HF, such as left ventricular hypertrophy (**111**) or previous MI (**112**). P mitrale may be present in mitral stenosis (**113**), whilst P pulmonale may be present in cor pulmonale (**114**). Wide bundle branch block (BBB) (**115**) is common in HF, and may suggest dyssynchronous cardiac contraction, which may improve with biventricular pacing.

An exercise ECG may occasionally induce cardiac arrhythmias (**116**).

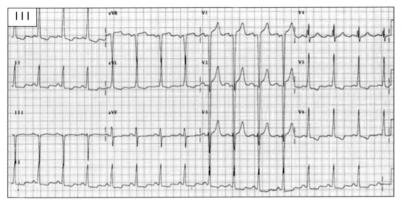

111 Electrocardiogram showing left ventricular hypertrophy; note large voltages in the precordial leads and ST depression laterally ('strain pattern').

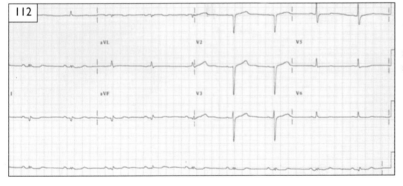

112 Electrocardiogram showing evidence of previous myocardial infarction; note q waves in leads III and aVF (inferior leads) and also in lead V I and lead V₂ (anterior leads).

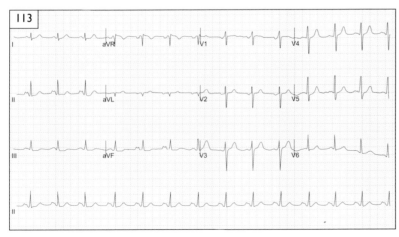

113 P mitrale (bifid p wave) indicating left atrial hypertrophy. In the absence of left ventricular hypertrophy, this may indicate mitral stenosis.

114 Electrocardiogram showing P pulmonale.

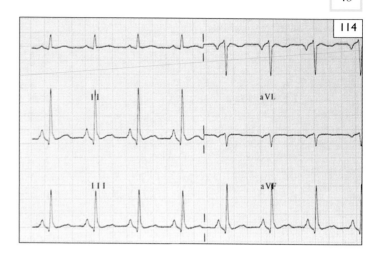

115 Electrocardiogram showing wide left bundle branch block. Atrial pacing spikes are also visible.

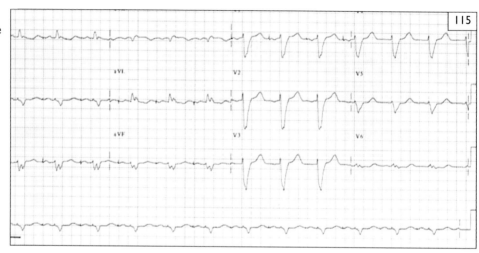

116 Electrocardiogram showing *torsade de pointes* with a heart rate of 189 bpm. This occurred at peak exercise.

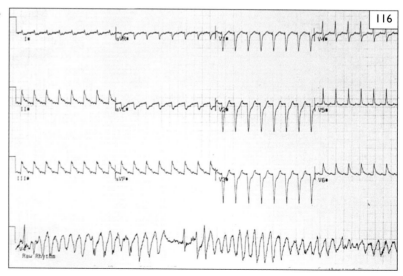

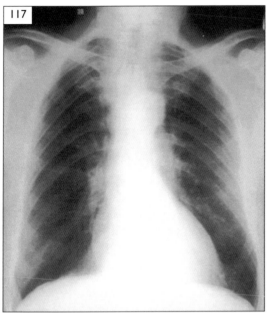

Chest X-ray

In patients with mild heart failure, the chest X-ray may be completely normal. An increase in the cardio-thoracic ratio (CTR) (>50%) may be seen, although this has poor sensitivity and specificity for the diagnosis of HF, and may be absent in acute HF due to MI. Increased CTR may be caused by left or right ventricular dilatation, hypertrophy of the left ventricle, or sometimes by large pericardial effusion (typically causing a 'globular' cardiac outline on X-ray) (117–121). Echocardiography is necessary to distinguish these causes. Occasionally, the chest X-ray may provide clues to the aetiology of HF; some examples include aortic calcification (122), mitral annular calcification (123), aortic dissection (124–126),

117–121 Chest X-ray showing gradually increasing cardiothoracic ratio and pulmonary oedema.

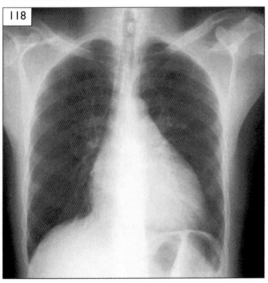

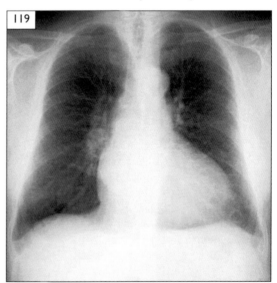

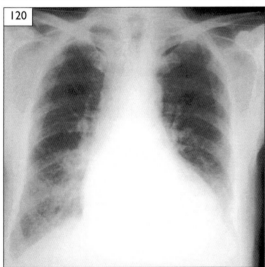

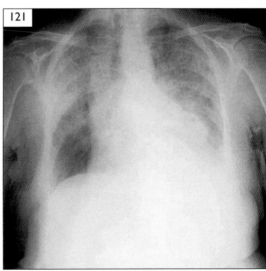

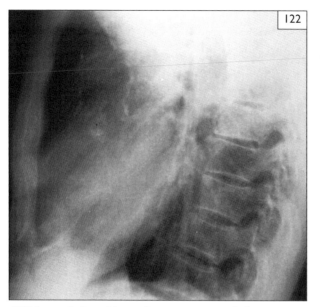

122 Lateral chest X-ray showing aortic calcification from previous aortitis, resulting in aortic regurgitation.

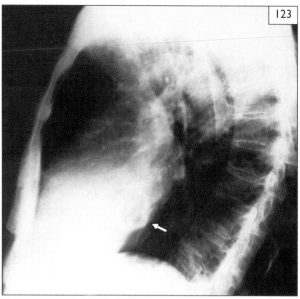

123 Lateral chest X-ray showing mitral annular calcifcation (arrow).

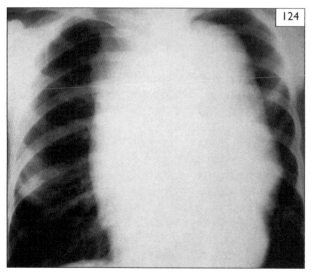

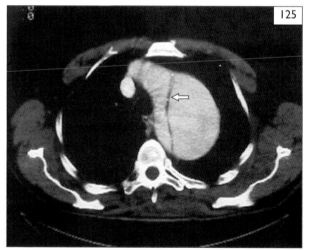

124–126 Aortic dissection. **124**: Chest X-ray; **125**: CT scan showing intimal flap (arrow); **126**: aortogram; true and false lumen with intimal flap (arrow).

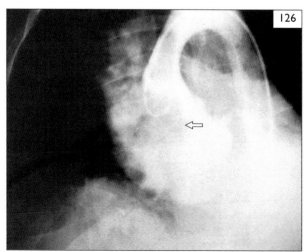

48

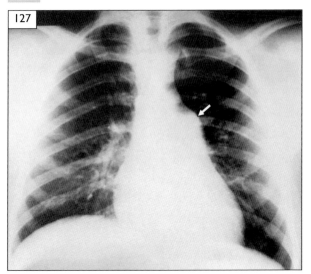

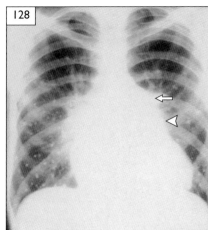

128 Mitral stenosis and pulmonary hypertension. Left atrial enlargement (arrowhead) and pulmonary artery dilatation (arrow).

127 Pulmonary stenosis – post stenotic dilatation of the pulmonary artery (arrow) and oligaemic lung fields.

pulmonary stenosis or pulmonary hypertension (**127, 128**), and aortic coarctation (**129**). A large left atrium in mitral stenosis may present with dysphagia, and evidence of indentation of the oesophagus may be seen on a barium swallow (**130-133**). An abnormal cardiac outline may be seen on chest X-ray where there is an LV aneurysm (**134, 135**). Pericardial calcification may be apparent in pericardial constriction (**136**).

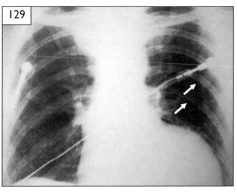

129 Coarctation of the aorta with rib notching (arrows) caused by collateral circulation.

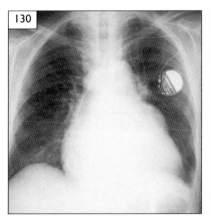

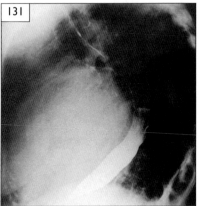

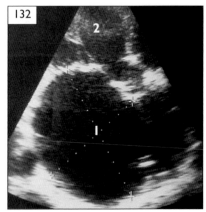

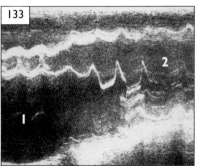

130–133 Giant left atrium. **130**: Marked left atrial enlargement; **131**: Barium swallow showing marked left atrial enlargement causing dysphagia by extrinsic oesophageal compression; **132**: Two-dimensional echocardiogram showing a giant left atrium (12 × 10 cm) in a patient with severe mitral regurgitation; **133**: M-mode echocardiogram showing giant left atrium. 1: left atrium; 2: left ventricle.

High quality films in the appropriate orientation are needed to assess the CTR accurately: the CTR may be exaggerated by antero-posterior X-ray films, or on a rotated film. In more advanced HF, the chest X-ray may show pleural effusions (which may be unilateral or bilateral), fluid in the transverse fissure of the right lung, upper lobe blood diversion (caused by vasoconstriction in the dependent, oedematous lung, and vasodilatation in the spared upper lobes), or signs of frank pulmonary congestion (137–142).

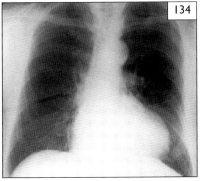
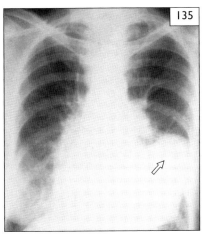
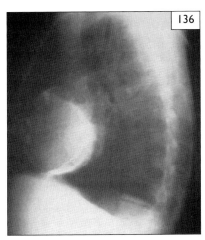

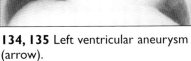

134, 135 Left ventricular aneurysm (arrow).

136 Extensive pericardial calcification in a patient with constrictive pericarditis.

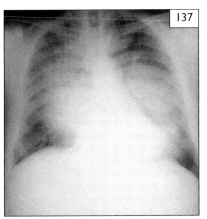
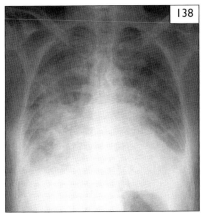
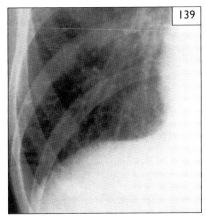

137–139 Acute pulmonary oedema. **137, 138**: bat's wing shadowing; **139**: Kerley B lines.

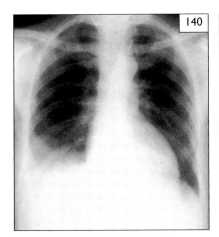
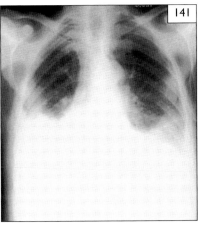
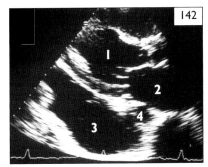

140–142 Pleural effusion. **140**: right pleural effusion; **141**: bilateral; **142**: pleural effusion on echocardiography. 1: left ventricle; 2: left atrium; 3: pleural effusion; 4: descending aorta.

In acute HF, the chest X-ray may also show signs of coexistent infection. It is important to be aware that pulmonary oedema may be noncardiac in origin (*Table 16*) and it is not possible to determine the cause from the chest X-ray alone. The chest X-ray may of course demonstrate a noncardiac cause of dyspnoea and, in addition, a patient with a normal chest X-ray and a normal ECG is very unlikely to have dyspnoea due to cardiac causes.

Blood tests

FULL BLOOD COUNT

Anaemia may exacerbate HF or, in the extremely anaemic patient, may be the underlying cause. Anaemia is common in HF, and is associated with a worse prognosis. Therefore, all patients with new or worsening HF should have a full blood count. In acute HF, a raised white cell count may point towards a coexistent infection.

CARDIAC ENZYMES AND CARDIAC TROPONINS

All patients presenting with acute HF should have serial cardiac enzymes and troponin estimation to exclude MI as the cause of their presentation. Patients with acute ischaemic HF often do not complain of chest pain, either because of silent ischaemia, or due to symptoms being masked by their acute shortness of breath. A high index of suspicion, guided by ECG and cardiac enzymes, is therefore necessary.

RENAL FUNCTION

Careful monitoring of renal function is essential in acute and chronic HF. In acute HF, poor cardiac output may lead to worsening renal function, a sign of poor prognosis. Medications such as diuretics and angiotenson-converting enzyme (ACE) inhibitors may adversely affect renal function, and the use of other medications such as digoxin may be hazardous in patients with impaired renal function. Hyponatraemia, due to neurohormonal activation, renal hypoperfusion, and medication is a marker of severe HF, and is a poor prognostic factor. Abnormalities of serum potassium predispose to malignant ventricular arrythmias. Hypokalaemia may occur as a result of loop diuretic therapy, while ACE inhibitors or spironolactone may result in hyperkalaemia, particularly when used in combination. Hypomagnesaemia often occurs in association with hypokalaemia, and also predisposes to ventricular arrhythmias. Hypomagnesaemia should be considered where hypokalaemia is severe or persistent, despite potassium replacement.

LIVER FUNCTION AND THYROID FUNCTION

Liver function tests are valuable to exclude hypoproteinaemia in patients with oedema of uncertain cause, although they may also be abnormal in advanced HF due to hepatic congestion. Hypothyroidism may cause lethargy and oedema, and hyperthyroidism may cause AF and high-output HF. Thyroid function tests are therefore recommended in HF, to exclude abnormalities of thyroid function and also because there is an association between thyroid dysfunction and ischaemic heart disease.

BRAIN NATRIURETIC PEPTIDE

The natriuretic peptide family is currently emerging as a useful investigative modality in HF. Brain natriuretic peptide (BNP), which is released from the ventricles in response to wall stretch, along with its N-terminal precursor (NT-ProBNP), appear to have the best specificity and sensitivity for HF (**143**). At present, the most widely accepted indications for the use of BNP or NT-ProBNP are:

- In the acutely breathless patient, where there is diagnostic difficulty. (High BNP has high positive predictive value for HF in this situation.)
- To exclude the diagnosis of HF in patients with no clinical signs. (Low BNP has high negative predictive value in this situation.)

Further study will be needed to determine if BNP or NT-ProBNP will be useful for the monitoring of

Table 16 Causes of pulmonary oedema
◇ Heart failure
◇ Renal failure
◇ Drugs, e.g. rosiglitazone
◇ Acute respiratory distress syndrome
◇ Altitude sickness
◇ Reexpansion pulmonary oedema (following rapid pleural drainage)
◇ Preeclampsia
◇ Fat embolism
◇ Amniotic fluid embolism
◇ Infections, e.g. malaria, Japanese B encephalitis
◇ Renal artery stenosis

progress in HF. It is very important to assess the BNP result in conjunction with clinical assessment of the patient, as unexpected values may occur occasionally, such as a very high BNP in a clinically stable patient. Additionally, BNP levels vary significantly from day to day within patients.

Echocardiography

Echocardiography is widely available, noninvasive, and can be performed with the patient sitting. It is therefore one of the most widely used techniques for objective assessment of cardiac structure and function (*Table 17*). Qualitative assessment of left ventricular

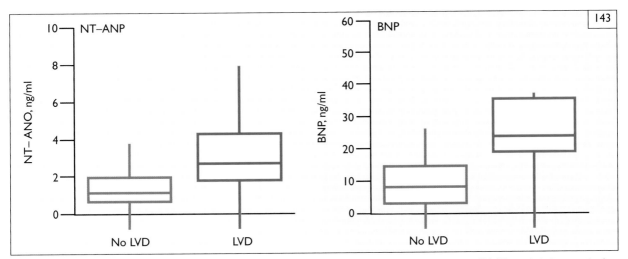

143 Correlation of serum atrial natriuretic peptide (ANP) and brain natriuretic peptide (BNP) with left ventricular dysfunction. Among 1252 subjects from the general population, median serum concentrations (boxes) of N-terminal ANP and BNP were significantly higher in those with symptomatic or asymptomatic left ventricular systolic dysfunction (LVD) as assessed with echocardiography. Vertical lines denote ranges of median serum concentrations. (From McDonagh TA, *et al. Lancet* 1998;**35**1:9.)

Table 17 Recommended data collection during echocardiographic examination

Minimum data set	Often also helpful	Sometimes applicable
Left ventricle		
M-mode		
LV chamber dimension at the level of the mitral leaflet tips	Claculation of fractional shortening	
Thickness of septum and posterior wall		Calculation of LV mass
Cross-sectional		
EF where possible, otherwise a qualitative description of LV systolic function	Cardiac output measurement by Doppler (or stroke distance)	Estimation of LV dP/dt$_{max}$ from the mitral regurgitant Doppler signal
Description of major wall motion abnormalities	Wall motion score	
	If LV function appears normal, a measurement of mitral valve and pulmonary vein inflow parameters may be useful	
Inspection of aortic, mitral, and tricuspid valves		
Colour flow search for regurgitant lesions		
Continuous wave estimation of valve gradients if valve appears abnormal	Continuity equation to assess AV area if output low and valve appears calcified	

AV: atrioventricular; EF: ejection fraction; LV: left ventricle.

(LV) function is possible in most patients (**144, 145**) and, in experienced hands, is of more value than the echocardiographic ejection fraction (EF) (stroke volume expressed as a percentage of end-diastolic volume, normally >50%), which has high inter- and intraobserver variability, and may not be obtained in patients with limited echocardiographic views. Worsening echocardiographic assessment of LV function correlates with worsening prognosis.

The echocardiogram provides information about the pattern of LV dysfunction. Ischaemic cardio-myopathy is typically associated with regional wall motion abnormalities, which may be described as hypokinetic (reduced wall movement and thickening during systole), akinetic (absent thickening although some movement may still occur in systole), or dyskinetic (paradoxical outward movement during systole). It is possible to calculate a wall motion score by applying these terms to different, standardized segments of myocardium (**146**). Dilated cardio-myopathy is associated with global, uniform LV dysfunction throughout all segments (**147**). Left ventricular hypertrophy in hypertensive heart disease is readily identified by echocardiography, and can be monitored to detect progression (or regression with treatment); Doppler in such patients may show reversed E to A ratio on the mitral inflow pattern, suggesting diastolic dysfunction (**148–150**).

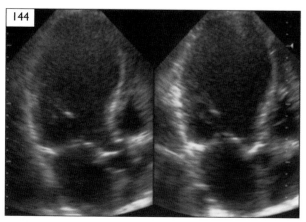

144 2D echocardiogram from a patient with previous myocardial infarction showing poor left ventricular function. The left image shows systole; the right diastole. Only the basal septum appears to move. The ejection fraction is at most 20%.

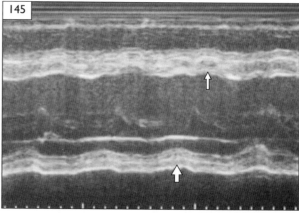

145 M-mode echocardiography showing poor left ventricular function, with little movement of the septum (small arrow) or posterior wall (large arrow).

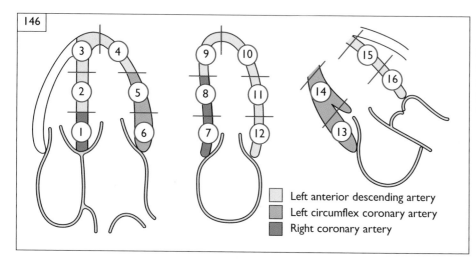

146 Diagrams showing the 16 regional wall segments and distribution of coronary perfusion. Left: apical four-chamber view; middle: apical two-chamber view; right: long-axis view.

Left anterior descending artery
Left circumflex coronary artery
Right coronary artery

147 M-mode and 2D
echocardiography showing
parasternal view in a patient
with dilated cardiomyopathy
– note thinned, immobile
septum and posterior wall.

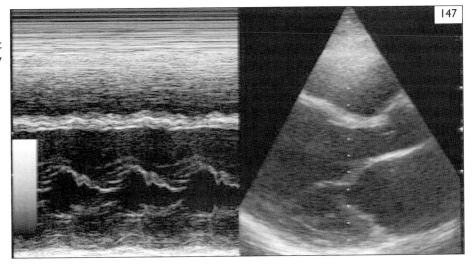

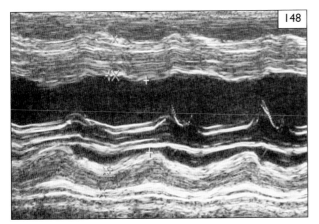

148 M-mode echocardiogram showing left ventricular
(LV) hypertrophy (septum 20 mm, LV posterior wall
12 mm).

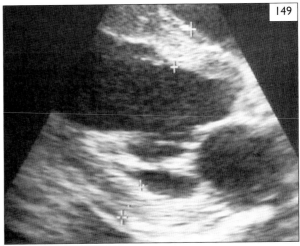

149 2D echocardiogram showing left ventricular
hypertrophy.

150 Pulse wave Doppler of mitral inflow,
showing reversed E:A ratio suggesting diastolic
dysfunction. 1: E wave – passive filling of left
ventricle; 2: A wave – atrial contraction.

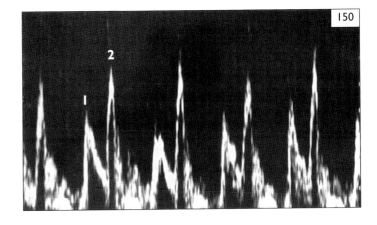

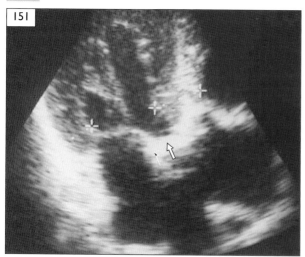

Stenotic or regurgitant valvular lesions are readily identified (**151–157**). 'Functional' mitral regurgitation, which occurs due to dilatation of the valvular annulus, is common in severe HF, and must be distinguished from structural mitral disease. Echocardiographic parameters of chamber size can be used to guide timing of valve replacement. The echocardiogram also provides information about atrial size (**158, 159**), presence of thrombus, and the function of the right heart (**160**).

151 2D echocardiogram showing severe calcification of the aortic valve (arrow).

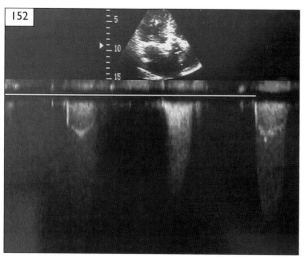

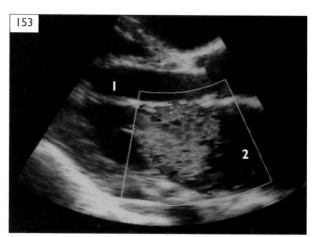

152 Continuous wave Doppler from the same patient as in **151** showing aortic stenosis, gradient 86 mmHg (11.5 kPa).

153 Congestive cardiomyopathy with an ejection fraction 15–20% showing severe mitral regurgitation on colour flow Doppler. 1: left ventricle; 2: left atrium.

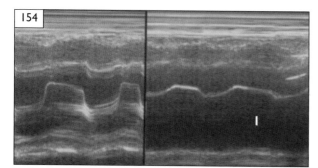

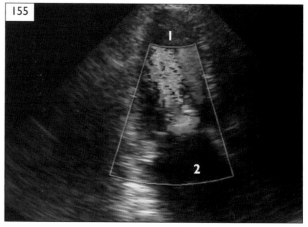

154 M-mode showing mitral stenosis (left part of image) and enlarged left atrium (right part of image). The patient was in atrial fibrillation. 1: left atrium.

155 Colour flow Doppler in mitral stenosis. 1: left ventricle; 2: left atrium.

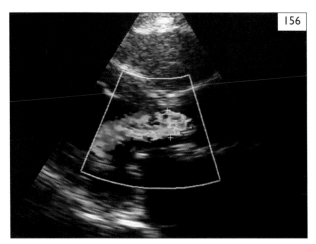

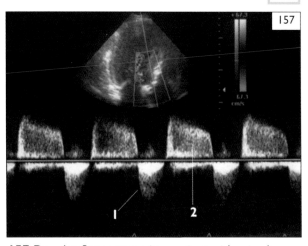

156 Colour flow Doppler showing severe aortic regurgitation. Measurement of regurgitant jet width is shown.

157 Doppler flow pattern in a patient with mixed aortic valve disease. 1: forward flow; 2: severe aortic regurgitation.

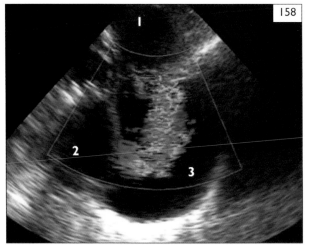

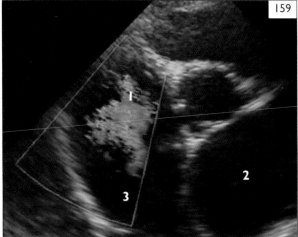

158, 159 Grossly enlarged right atrium and severe tricuspid regurgitation in a patient with a prosthetic mitral valve. 1: right ventricle; 2: left atrium; 3: right atrium.

160 Severe tricuspid regurgitation in a patient with pulmonary hypertension due to chronic obstructive pulmonary disease. The patient is in atrial fibrillation.

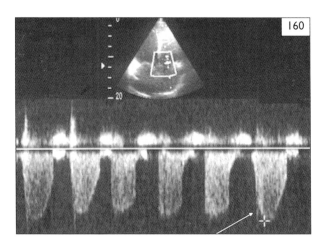

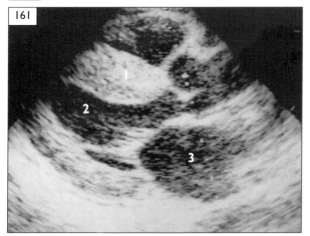

161 Echocardiogram in a patient with pseudo left ventricular hypertrophy due to amyloid. 1: interventricular septum; 2: left ventricle; 3: left atrium.

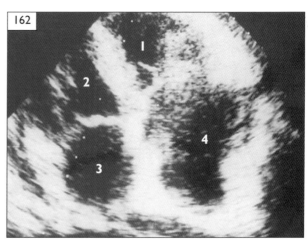

162 Echocardiogram in a patient with restrictive cardiomyopathy due to amyloid. 1: left ventricle; 2:right ventricle; 3: right atrium; 4: left atrium.

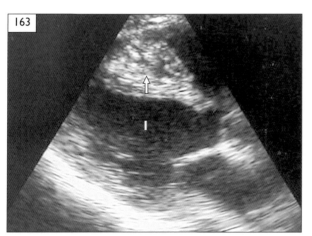

163 Echocardiogram showing hypertrophic cardiomyopathy – note asymmetrical septal hypertrophy (arrow). 1: left ventricle.

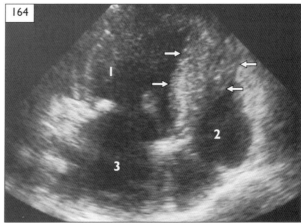

164 Two-dimensional echocardiogram (4 chamber view) showing mid apical hypertrophic cardiomyopathy (arrows). 1: left ventricle; 2: right ventricle; 3: left atrium.

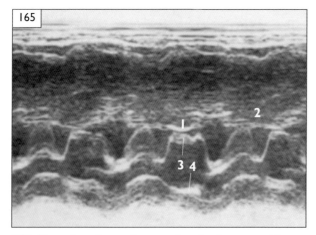

165 M-mode echocardiogram showing hypertrophic cardiomyopathy with systolic anterior motion of the mitral valve (1). 2: interventricular septum; 3: anterior mitral valve leaflet; 4: posterior mitral valve leaflet.

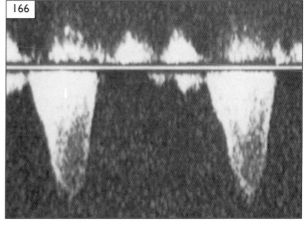

166 Doppler scan showing hypertrophic cardiomyopathy with mid systolic maximal velocity of the mitral regurgitation jet (1).

Other rarer cases of HF may be shown by echocardiography. Examples include amyloid heart disease (**161, 162**) and hypertrophic cardiomyopathy (**163–166**).

The optimal method for echocardiographic assessment of diastolic function has not yet been established. The commonest methods involve assessment of mitral flow patterns using pulsed Doppler studies (**150**), but these methods are limited by dependence upon pre- and afterload conditions. Newer assessment methods under investigation include tissue Doppler mitral valve ring motion analysis, and colour Doppler flow. As discussed in Chapter 1, there is controversy whether diastolic dysfunction can be diagnosed simply in those with symptoms and signs of HF but preserved systolic function, or whether objective evidence of abnormalities of the above parameters is necessary.

Nuclear scanning
Multi-gated ventriculography (MUGA), a noninvasive radionuclide method in which scanning is synchronized with the ECG ('gated'), provides measurement of the EF, which is less operator-dependent than echocardiography. Images may also be obtainable in patients who are poor echocardiography subjects. Equilibrium ventriculography involves labelling and studying a sample of the subject's blood with technetium-99m, whereas first-pass ventriculography involves studying the passage of a bolus of tracer using gamma cameras. Nuclear imaging may also be used to detect ischaemia (**167**), as well as 'stunned' or 'hibernating' myocardium. However, the techniques are not as widely available as echocardiography, are more expensive, and involve a significant radiation dose.

Magnetic resonance imaging
Magnetic resonance imaging (MRI) can provide extremely clear cardiac images, and is particularly useful in patients with poor echocardiographic visualization of the heart. MRI allows visualization from almost any angle, including reproduction of the commonly used echocardiographic views. MRI has low interobserver variation for LV function, and is regarded by some as the preferred method to assess LV mass and LVEF. MRI appears to be a promising tool in the identification of hibernating myocardium. MRI requires patients to lie flat, and also to breath-hold on command, which some patients may find difficult. Additionally, some patients find the scanner claustrophobic. MRI cannot be performed in patients with pacemakers or other metallic implants, but appears to be safe in those with various coronary stents *in situ* especially after endothelialization of the stent over the weeks postdeployment. Cardiac MRI may demonstrate other abnormalities, including constrictive pericarditis (**168**) and coarctation of the aorta.

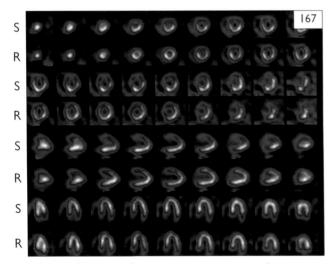

167 Nuclear scan demonstrating anterior ischaemia with partial reversibility. S: stress; R: rest.

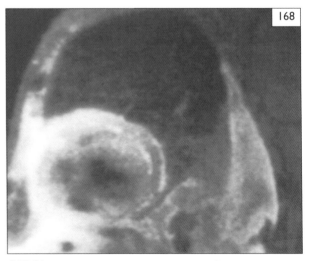

168 Magnetic resonance imaging scan showing tuberculous constrictive pericarditis.

Cardiac catheterization

Ischaemic heart disease is the commonest cause of HF in the western world. Patients with recurring symptoms of ischaemia, objective evidence of reversible ischaemia, or evidence of hibernating segments of myocardium should be considered for angiography and, where indicated, revascularization. LV angiography also provides an alternative method of assessing LV structure and function (**169, 170**) and mitral regurgitation (**171**), including end-diastolic pressure (**172, 173**). Right heart catheterization allows assessment of oxygen saturation (useful in the detection of intracardiac shunts), as well as right-sided pressure and pulmonary artery wedge pressure (**174–176**). Pulmonary angiography may demonstrate pulmonary emboli (**177**). Cardiac catheterization and myocardial biopsy can be useful in cases of diagnostic difficulty.

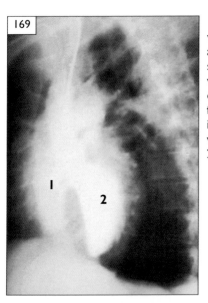

169 Left ventricular angiogram showing a large ventricular septal defect and free flow of contrast into the right ventricle (1). 2: left ventricle.

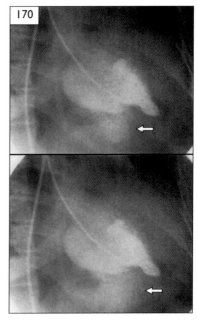

170 Left ventricular pseudoaneurysm following myocardial infarction and chronic ventricular rupture. Note leak of contrast from the left ventricular cavity to the pericardial space (arrow).

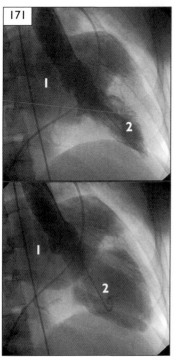

171 Left ventricular angiogram in gross mitral regurgitation systolic frame (top); diastolic frame (bottom). 1: left atrium; 2: left ventricle.

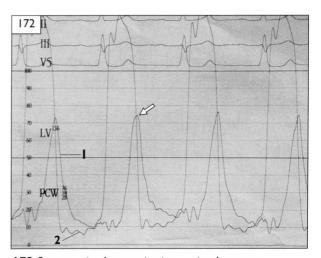

172 Severe mitral regurgitation – simultaneous pulmonary wedge pressure (1) and left ventricular diastolic pressure (2). V wave 75 mmHg (10 kPa) (arrow).

173 Mixed mitral valve disease, stenosis > regurgitation – simultaenous pulmonary wedge pressure (1) and left ventricular diastolic pressure (2). End-diastolic gradient (3) 12 mmHg (1.6 kPa).

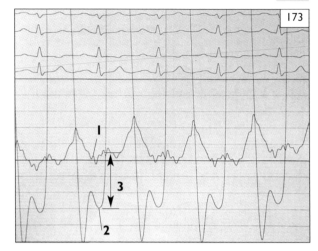

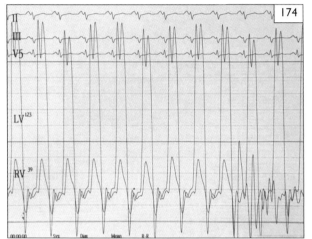

174 Contrictive pericarditis – simultaneous right and left ventricular tracings showing near identical diastolic pressures with a dip and plateau appearance.

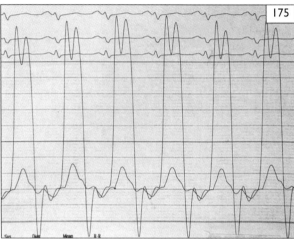

175 Constrictive pericarditis – simultaneous pulmonary artery and left ventricular tracings showing near identical diastolic pressures.

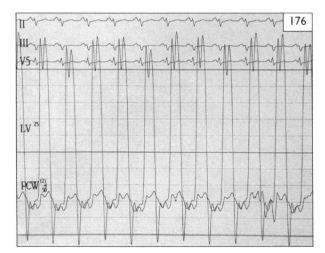

176 Constrictive pericarditis – simultaneous pulmonary artery wedge and left ventricular tracings showing near identical diastolic pressures.

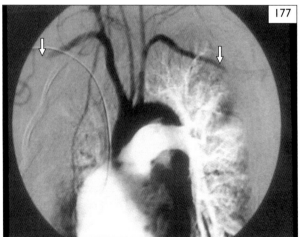

177 Late phase pulmonary angiogram showing absent right pulmonary artery due to acute right-sided pulmonary embolus and bilateral subclavian artery emboli (arrows) in a patient with vasculitis.

Some typical cardiac catheterization findings are worthy of mention. In hypertrophic cardiomyopathy (178, 179), cardiac catheterization may show a mid cavity gradient, or sometimes a postectopic gradient or gradient with valsalva (180–182). In aortic stenosis, a slow rising pulse on the aortic trace as well as a pressure gradient may be shown on 'pull back' of the catheter from the LV cavity to the aorta (183, 184).

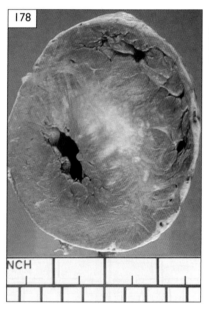

178 Pathology specimen of hypertrophic cardiomyopathy.

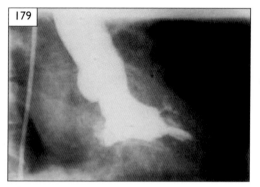

179 Cardiac catheterization showing hypertrophic cardiomyopathy (apical left ventricular cavity obliteration) and mitral valve prolapse.

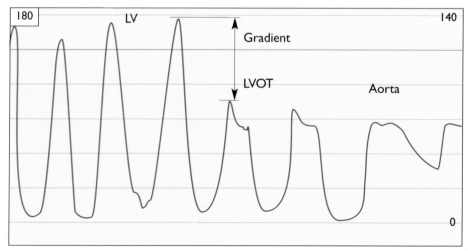

180 Hypertrophic cardiomyopathy and left ventricular outflow tract (LVOT) gradient. LV: left ventricle.

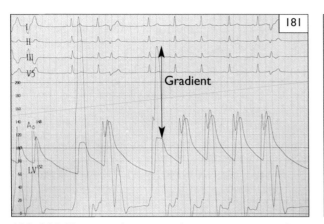

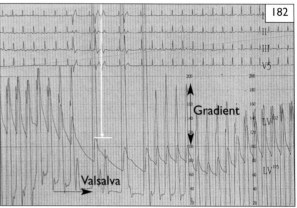

181, 182 Electrocardiogram and pressure tracings showing hypertrophic cardiomyopathy. **181**: postectopic gradient; **182**: valsalva manoeuvre; no apparent gradient at rest, gradient apparent during and following valsalva manoeuvre.

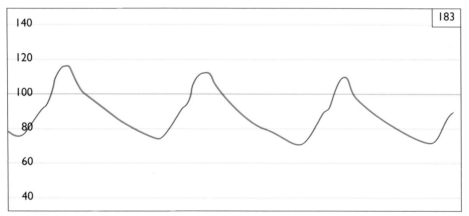

183 Aortic stenosis; slow rising aortic pressure trace.

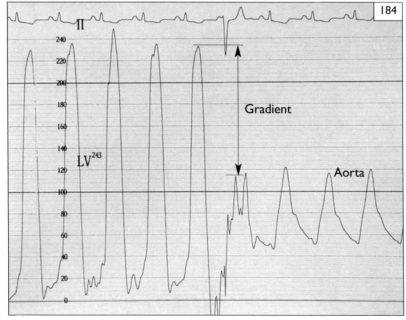

184 Pressure trace on pullback from left ventricle (LV) to aorta showing severe aortic stenosis.

In contrast, aortic regurgitation is associated with a wide pulse pressure on the aortic trace (185, 186). Coarctation of the aorta gives a typical appearance on the aortogram (187, 188). The aortogram may show renal artery stenosis, which is a rare cause of flash pulmonary oedema (189).

Exercise testing

The New York Heart Association (NYHA) classification stratifies patients according to exercise capacity, but is clearly a relatively crude tool. More detailed information regarding exercise capacity and gas exchange can be obtained from formal exercise testing with assessment of peak oxygen uptake ($VO2_{max}$). Exercise may be performed either on a treadmill or by bicycle; $VO2_{max}$ has been shown to be 10–20% higher when assessed with treadmill exercise. A normal $VO2_{max}$ virtually excludes the diagnosis of HF. $VO2_{max}$ correlates well with maximum cardiac output, and has been shown in several studies to predict outcome in HF better than other parameters such as EF.

Exercise testing has been shown to be safe in patients with significant HF, with a low incidence of arrhythmias or other adverse effects. Limitations include lack of

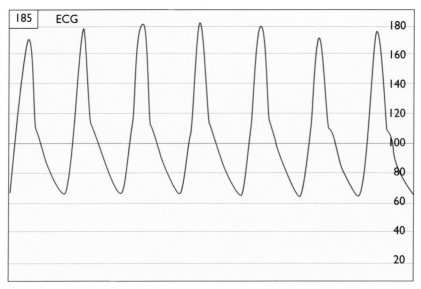

185 Aortic pressure trace in aortic regurgitation showing wide pulse pressure.

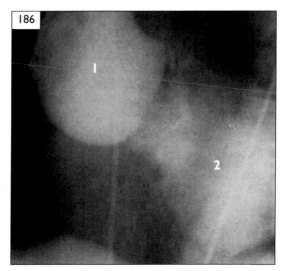

186 Aortic regurgitation due to Marfan syndrome – note the 'onion bulb' shape to the aortic root (1). 2: left ventricle.

availability, and practical difficulties with patients who are poorly mobile or unused to bicycle or treadmill exercise. Results are dependent upon the patient exercising to their anaerobic threshold, which is partly dependent upon patient motivation.

Heart rate variability
Heart rate variability (HRV) is a term used to describe a variety of indices calculated from either short-term (2–20 minutes) or 24-hour ECG recordings, which quantify the beat-to-beat changes in heart rate which occur in normal individuals. A variety of variables can be obtained from time-domain and frequency-domain analyses of HRV. Various disease processes and drugs affect the indices of HRV. Notably, in HF HRV is significantly reduced compared to controls. Reduced HRV is superior to LVEF for prediction of sudden death or ventricular tachycardia post-MI. The UK Heart Failure Evaluation and Assessment of Risk Trial (UK-HEART) found reduced 24-hour SDNN (standard deviation of R-R intervals) to be a better predictor of death due to progressive HF than conventional clinical criteria. Retrospective analysis of the Veterans Affairs' Survival Trial of Antiarrhythmic Therapy in Congestive Heart Failure found that each increase of 10 ms in SDNN conferred a 20% decrease in risk of mortality and, further, that patients with SDNN in the lowest quartile had a significantly increased risk of sudden death.

Importantly, several drug therapies including ACE inhibitors, β-blockers, and spironolactone, which reduce mortality in HF, also increase HRV. These drug therapies reduce sudden death in HF, and it has been suggested that this may be due to their effects on HRV. However, other drugs which increase HRV (such as scopolamine) have not been shown to reduce mortality in HF and, therefore, it is not clear whether increasing HRV directly leads to decreased mortality.

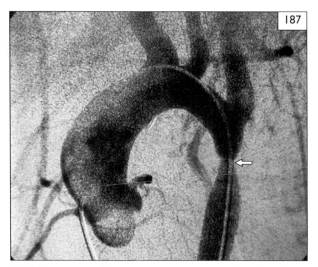

187 Aortogram showing coarctation just distal to the left subclavian artery (arrow).

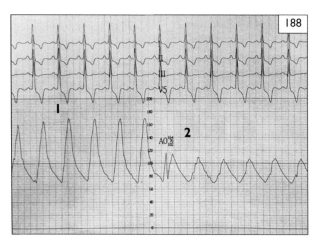

188 Aortic pressure tracing in a patient with coarctation. 1: ascending aorta; 2: descending aorta.

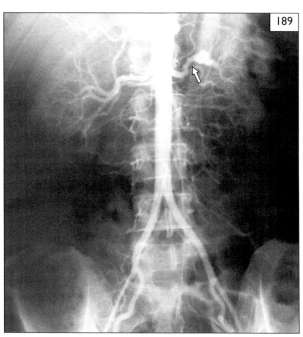

189 Renal artery stenosis (arrow) due to fibromuscular dysplasia additionally affecting the femoral arteries.

Further reading

ACC/AHA guidelines for the evaluation and management of chronic heart failure in the adult: a report of the American College of Cardiology/American Heart Association Task Force on practice Guidelines. 2001. American College of Cardiology Website. Available at: http://www.acc.org/clinical/guidelines/failure/hf_index.htm

Corra U, Mezzani A, Bosimini E, Giannuzzi P. Cardiopulmonary exercise testing and prognosis in chronic heart failure: a prognosticating algorithm for the individual patient. *Chest* 2004;**126**(3):942–950.

Dao Q, Krishnaswamy P, Kazanegra R, *et al*. Utility of B-type natriuretic peptide in the diagnosis of congestive heart failure in an urgent-care setting. *J. Am. Coll. Cardiol.* 2001;**37**:379–385.

Frenneaux MP. Autonomic changes in patients with heart failure and in postmyocardial infarction patients. *Heart* 2004;**90**(11):1248–1255.

Hobbs FDR, Davis RC, Roalfe AK, *et al*. Reliability of N-terminal pro-brain natriuretic peptide assay in diagnosis of heart failure: cohort study in representative and high risk community populations. *BMJ* 2002;**324**:1498–1500.

Zile MR, Brutsaert DL. New concepts in diastolic dysfunction and diastolic heart failure: Part I. Diagnosis, prognosis, and measurements of diastolic function. *Circulation* 2002;**105**:1387–1393.

Chapter five
Drugs affecting the renin– angiotensin–aldosterone system and diuretics

Introduction
In the UK, the recent National Institute for Clinical Excellence (NICE) guidelines provide a useful algorithm for the treatment of heart failure (HF) due to systolic dysfunction (**190**). The drug treatment of HF is designed to alleviate symptoms and improve

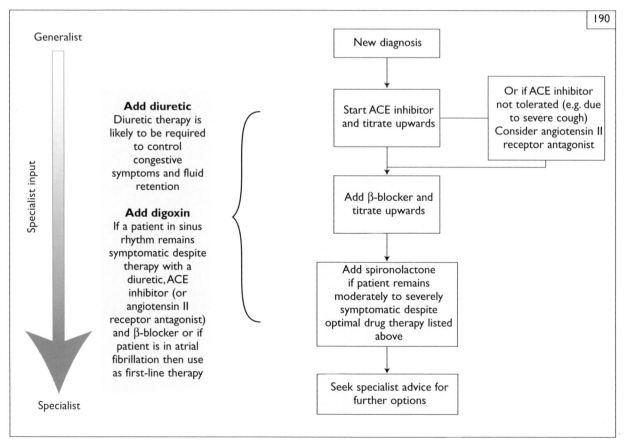

Generalist

Specialist input

Specialist

Add diuretic
Diuretic therapy is likely to be required to control congestive symptoms and fluid retention

Add digoxin
If a patient in sinus rhythm remains symptomatic despite therapy with a diuretic, ACE inhibitor (or angiotensin II receptor antagonist) and β-blocker or if patient is in atrial fibrillation then use as first-line therapy

New diagnosis

Start ACE inhibitor and titrate upwards

Or if ACE inhibitor not tolerated (e.g. due to severe cough) Consider angiotensin II receptor antagonist

Add β-blocker and titrate upwards

Add spironolactone if patient remains moderately to severely symptomatic despite optimal drug therapy listed above

Seek specialist advice for further options

190 Algorithm for the pharmacological treatment of symptomatic heart failure due to left ventricular systolic dysfunction. Patients should be treated with the following drugs (if tolerated and not contraindicated) and in the sequence indicated. ACE: angiotensin-converting enzyme. NB:
◇ Diuretics is first-line therapy when a patient presents with acute pulmonary oedema.
◇ Left-hand margin arrow indicates the increasing likelihood of the need for specialist input.

prognosis. The various drugs employed have different mechanisms of action, varying effects (*Table 18*), and can be introduced at different stages of HF (**191**).

This chapter will focus upon drugs that interfere with the renin–angiotensin–aldosterone system, and diuretics.

Angiotensin-converting enzyme inhibitors
The introduction of angiotensin-converting enzyme (ACE) inhibitors in the 1980s has probably been the most important pharmacological weapon in the treatment of left ventricular systolic dysfunction (*Table 19*). The benefits of these drugs in improving both mortality and morbidity in all grades of HF have been repeatedly demonstrated in several large, randomized controlled trials. Indeed, Framingham data have revealed improving survival of patients with HF, in keeping with increasingly widespread use of ACE inhibitors.

Table 18 Pharmacological therapy

	Improved symptoms	Decreased mortality	Prevention of chronic HF	Neurohormonal control
Diuretics	Yes	?	?	No
Digoxin	Yes	=	Minimal	Yes
Inotropes	Yes	Increased	?	No
Vasodilators (nitrates)	Yes	Yes	?	No
ACE inhibitors	Yes	Yes+	Yes	Yes+
Other neurohormonal drugs	Yes	+/-	?	Yes+

ACE: angiotensin-converting enzyme; HF: heart failure; Yes+: large response.

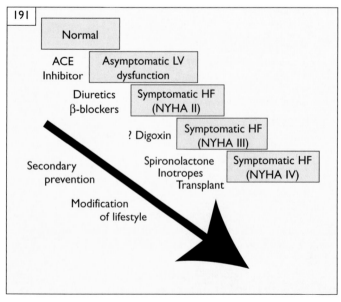

191 Treatment according to the degree of heart failure. Patients with asymptomatic ventricular dysfunction should receive angiotensin-converting enzyme inhibitors (ACEI). In the presence of symptoms of heart failure, diuretics or neurohormonal inhibitors should be added. The use of digoxin remains controversial. In more advanced stages in the presence of poorly controlled symptoms, newer drugs can be tried, reserving the inotropes for patients whose symptoms are uncontrollable with other medication. Secondary prevention and assisting the patient in adapting to their limitations should also be addressed. EF: ejection fraction; HF: heart failure; LV: left ventricular; NYHA: New York Heart Association.

Table 19 Practical recommendations on the use of angiotenson-converting enzyme (ACE) inhibitors

Which ACE inhibitor and what dose?

Licensed ACE inhibitor	Starting dose (mg)	Target dose (mg)
Captopril	6.25 TID	50–100 TID
Cilazapril*	0.5 OD	1–2.5 OD
Enalapril	2.5 BID	10–20 BID
Fosinopril*	10 OD	40 OD
Lisinopril	2.5–5.0 OD	30–35 OD
Perindopril*	2.0 OD	4.0 OD
Quinapril*	2.5–5.0 OD	10–20 OD
Ramipril	2.5 OD	5.0 BID or 10.0 OD

* Target dose based on manufacturer's recommendation rather than large outcome study.

How to use
◇ Start with a low dose (see above)
◇ Seek specialist advice where the patient is on high dose of a loop diuretic (e.g. frusemide [furosemide] 80 mg)
◇ Double dose at not less than 2 week intervals
◇ Aim for target dose (see above) or, failing that, the highest tolerated dose
◇ Remember some ACE inhibitor is better than none
◇ Monitor blood electrolytes (in particular potassium), urea, creatinine, and blood pressure
◇ When to stop up-titration/down-titration: see Problem solving

Advice to patient
◇ Explain expected benefits
◇ Treatment is given to improve symptoms, to prevent worsening of heart failure, and to increase survival
◇ Symptoms improve within a few weeks to a few months of starting treatment
◇ Advise patients to report principal adverse effects (e.g. dizziness/symptomatic hypotension, cough)

Problem solving
◇ Asymptomatic low blood pressure does not usually require any change in therapy

Symptomatic hypotension
◇ If dizziness, light headedness, and/or confusion and a low blood pressure consider discontinuing nitrates, calcium channel blockers and other vasodilators
◇ If no signs/symptoms of congestion consider reducing diuretic dose
◇ If these measures do not solve the problem seek specialist advice

Cough
◇ Cough is common in patients with chronic heart failure, many of whom have smoking-related lung disease
◇ Cough is also a symptom of pulmonary oedema which should be excluded when a new or worsening cough develops
◇ ACE inhibitor-induced cough rarely requires treatment discontinuation
◇ If the patient develops a troublesome cough which interferes with sleep and is likely to be caused by an ACE inhibitor, consider substituting an angiotensin II receptor antagonist

Worsening renal function
◇ Some rise in urea, creatinine and K^+ is to be expected after initiation of an ACE inhibitor. If the increase is small and asymptomatic no action is necessary
◇ An increase in creatinine up to 50% above baseline, or to 200 µmol/l (2.3 mg/dl), whichever is the smaller, is acceptable
◇ An increase in K^+ to ≤5.9 mmol/l (5.9 mEq/l) is acceptable
◇ If urea, creatinine, or K^+ do rise excessively, consider stopping concomitant nephrotoxic drugs (e.g. NSAIDs), nonessential vasodilators (e.g. calcium antagonists, nitrates), K^+ supplements/retaining agents (triamterine, amiloride) and, if no signs of congestion, reducing the dose of diuretic
◇ If greater rises in creatinine or K^+ than those outlined above persist, despite adjustment of concomitant medication, the dose of the ACE inhibitor should be halved and blood chemistry rechecked. If there is still an unsatisfactory response, specialist advice should be sought
◇ If K^+ rises to ≥6.0 mmol/l (6.0 mEq/l) or creatinine increases by >100% or to >350 µmol/l (4.0 mg/dl) the dose of ACE inhibitor should be stopped and specialist advice sought
◇ Blood electrolytes should be monitored closely until K^+ and creatinine concentrations are stable

NB: It is very rarely necessary to stop an ACE inhibitor and clinical deterioration is likely if treatment is withdrawn. Ideally, specialist advice should be sought before treatment is discontinued. ACE: angiotensin-converting enzyme inhibitor; NSAID: nonsteroidal anti-inflammatory drug. (From McMurray JJV, *et al. Eur. J. Heart Fail.* 2001;**3**:495–502.)

MECHANISM OF ACTION

ACE inhibitors attenuate the activation of the renin–angiotensin–aldosterone system (RAAS) seen to occur in HF (see Chapter 3). Their benefits are related, in part, to reduced production of angiotensin II (**192**). This diminishes the resulting vasoconstriction (and increased systemic vascular resistance) and aldosterone-related sodium retention, as well as inhibiting further sympathetic activation. Furthermore, angiotensin II-mediated myocyte hypertrophy and apoptosis, which may contribute to cardiac remodelling, are also reduced.

In addition to their impact on the RAAS, ACE inhibitors also affect the kallikrein-kinin system (**192**). One of the products of this axis, bradykinin, appears to counteract certain angiotensin II-mediated effects, resulting in beneficial vasodilatory and natriuretic effects. Bradykinin is degraded into inactive fragments by ACE. Thus, this nonspecific enzyme inhibition of at least two important pathophysiological pathways may result in the clinical benefits seen.

CLINICAL BENEFITS

Heart failure

The now undisputed survival benefits of ACE inhibition were first demonstrated in the COoperative North Scandinavian ENalapril SUrvival Study (CONSENSUS) in 1987 (**193**). Patients with severe (New York Heart Association [NYHA] functional class IV) HF were randomized to treatment with either enalapril or placebo, and were followed up for 20 months. At this point, a striking reduction in mortality of 27% was apparent, mainly by reducing deaths from progressive HF. Subsequently, in the Studies Of Left Ventricular Dysfunction-treatment trial (SOLVD-T), enalapril was seen to reduce both mortality (**194**) and hospitalization for HF in patients with milder HF (NYHA II–III). After 12 years of follow-up, enalapril was still seen to confer a survival advantage, with median survival greater by 9 months over placebo (for patients in both treatment and prevention arms).

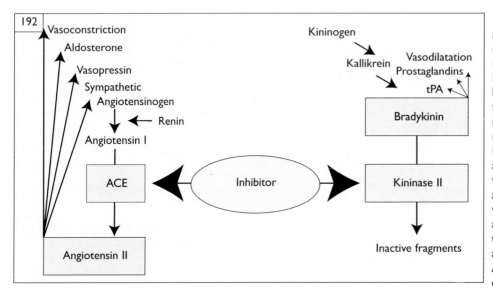

192 Mechanism of action of angiotensin-converting enzyme (ACE) inhibitors. ACE inhibitors competitively block the enzyme that transforms angiotensin I into angiotensin II. The reduction in angiotensin II levels explains the arteriovenous vasodilatatory action, as angiotensin II is a potent vasoconstrictor that augments sympathetic tone in the arteriovenous system. Additionally, angiotensin causes vasopressin release and produces sodium and water retention, both through a direct renal effect and through liberation of aldosterone. Since the converting enzyme has a similar structure to kininase II that degrades bradykinin, ACE inhibitors increase kinin levels that are potent vasodilators (E2 and F2) and increase release of fibrinolytic substances such as tissue plasminogen activator (tPA).

193 Angiotensin-converting enzyme (ACE) inhibitors and survival (CONSENSUS). Prolonged administration of ACE inhibitors reduces mortality in symptomatic heart failure. The first study to demonstrate this effect was CONSENSUS I. This graph shows the cumulative mortality curves of the treatment and placebo groups in this randomized, double-blind trial. The study analyzed the effect of enalapril on prognosis of 253 patients with class IV heart failure, who also

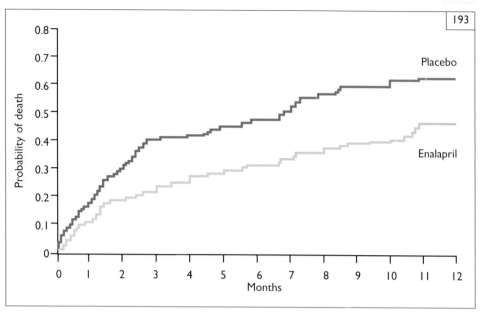

received digitalis, diuretics, and conventional vasodilators. At the end of 6 months of treatment, there was a clear-cut improvement in functional class, a reduction in the need for medications, and a 40% reduction in mortality ($p<0.002$). After 12 months, the mortality reduction was 31% ($p<0.001$). Nonetheless, there were no differences in the incidence of sudden death between the two groups, or in the subgroup that received other conventional vasodilators. Another characteristic of this study was variability of the dose that was used for each patient (adjusted for tolerance and symptoms): 2.5–40 mg/day. This aspect shows the importance of individualized treatment for heart failure patients. (From CONSENSUS Trial Study Group. *N. Engl. J. Med.* 1987;**316**:1429.)

194 Angiotensin-converting enzyme (ACE) inhibitors and survival (SOLVD). Mortality curves in patients with clinical heart failure in the SOLVD treatment study. In this study, 2569 symptomatic heart failure patients with ejection fractions <35% (90% in functional class II–III) were randomized to receive enalapril (n=1285) or placebo (n=1284). Mortality over a 41-month follow-up period was 39.7% in the enalapril arm and 35.2% in the placebo arm ($p<0.004$). The mortality reduction was chiefly mediated through less progression of heart failure; deaths due to arrhythmia were not reduced. Additionally, the enalapril group required fewer hospitalizations for heart failure. (From SOLVD (Treatment). *N. Engl. J. Med.* 1991;**325**:293.)

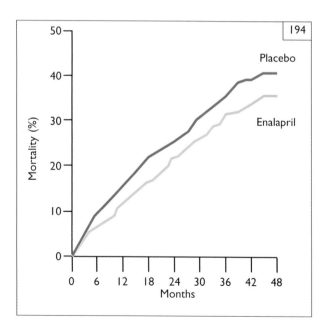

The morbidity benefit was also highlighted by the Quinapril Heart Failure Trial, which assessed the need for additional treatments in patients with mild–moderate HF, who either continued or discontinued taking quinapril (**195**).

Asymptomatic left ventricular dysfunction
The SOLVD trial had a prevention arm, designed to study the effects of ACE inhibition upon mortality and morbidity in over 4000 patients with left ventricular ejection fraction (LVEF) <35%, but no symptoms. This trial did not reveal significant mortality benefit of enalapril after 4 years of follow-up (**196**), but did delay the development of HF, and reduced hospitalizations for HF by 20%.

Left ventricular systolic dysfunction (LVSD) postmyocardial infarction
Several studies have demonstrated mortality benefit of ACE inhibition after myocardial infarction (MI), irrespective of the presence of symptoms of HF (*Tables 20, 21*). The Survival And Ventricular Enlargement (SAVE) Study recruited asymptomatic patients with ejection fraction <40% post-MI, and compared survival in those treated with captopril or placebo (**197**). Treatment with captopril was associated with a mortality reduction of 19%, reduced risk of hospitalization for HF, and a reduced risk of subsequent MI of 25%. In contrast, the Acute Infarction Ramipril Efficacy (AIRE) Study, another randomized placebo-controlled trial, recruited symptomatic patients, but those treated with ramipril

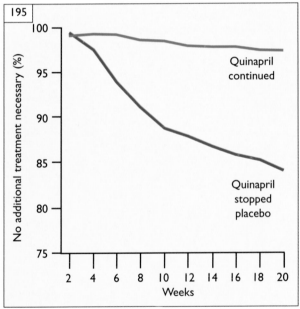

195 Angiotensin-converting enzyme (ACE) inhibitors and effect on symptoms. The effect of discontinuation of quinapril therapy on patients with class II–III heart failure in the Quinapril Heart Failure Trial is shown. At 20 weeks of treatment, the group whose quinapril treatment was terminated (n=110) had increased symptoms compared to the group who continued to receive quinapril therapy (n=114). The latter group maintained a stable functional status. This study, whose design was similar to PROVED and RADIANCE, again demonstrates the efficacy of ACE inhibitors in the treatment of heart failure. (From Pflugfelder PW, et al. J. Am. Coll. Cardiol. 1993;**22**:1557.)

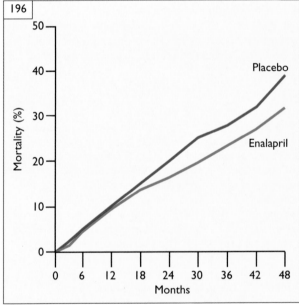

196 Angiotensin-converting enzyme (ACE) inhibitors and survival in asymptomatic ventricular dysfunction. Mortality curves in patients with asymptomatic ventricular dysfunction in the SOLVD study. This study compared the effect of enalapril (n=2111) versus placebo (n=2117) in 4228 asymptomatic patients with ejection fraction <35% who were previously untreated. Overall mortality was similar in both groups (15.8% versus 14.8%, NS), but in the enalapril arm a reduction in development of clinical symptoms of heart failure or need for hospitalization was seen. Once again, patients with the lowest ejection fractions were those who benefited the most from therapy. (From SOLVD Investigators. N. Engl. J. Med. 1992;**327**:685.)

Table 20 Angiotensin-converting enzyme inhibitors in postmyocardial infarction

Study	Population	Premature deaths prevented per 1000 patients treated	Study medication and dose
AIRE	Clinical or radiological evidence of LV failure	12	Ramipril 5 mg BID
SAVE	Asymptomatic LV dysfunction	45	Captopril 50 mg TID
ISIS 4, GISSI 3, CCS-1, SMILE	Unselected normotensives	5–8	Captopril 50 mg BID Captopril 12.5 mg TID Zofenopril 60 mg/day

LV: left ventricular. (For Trials see Appendix A.)

Table 21 Angiotensin-converting enzyme (ACE) inhibitors in postinfarction survival

	ACE inhibitor	Benefit	Patient selection
ISIS-4	Captopril	5/5 week	All with AMI
GISSI-3	Lisinopril	0.8/6 week	All with AMI
SAVE	Captopril	4.2/3.5 year	EF <40 asymptomatic
SMILE	Zofenopril	4.1/1 year	Anterior AMI
TRACE	Trandolapril	7.6/3 year	Ventricular dysfunction/ clinical chronic HF, EF <35
AIRE	Ramipril	6/1 year	Clinical chronic HF

AMI: acute myocardial infarction; EF: ejection fraction; HF: heart failure. The results of the various studies that have compared ACE inhibitors with placebo in the postmyocardial infarction (MI) setting have differing results. Nonetheless, the benefit obtained in each study correlates with the degree of ventricular dysfunction of the selected patients. In this table, the difference in mortality over time is seen in absolute terms: lives saved /100 patients treated = % mortality in placebo group - % mortality in ACE inhibitor group/follow-up time. Even though the studies demonstrated statistically significant differences between placebo and ACE inhibitor therapy, the benefit of treatment is minimal in low-risk patients, probably not justifying its routine use in every post-MI patient (ISIS-4 and GISSI-3). Benefits are moderate in patients with higher risk (asymptomatic ventricular dysfunction) (SAVE and SMILE), and maximal in patients with severe ventricular dysfunction or clinical heart failure (TRACE and AIRE). (For Trials see Appendix A.)

197 Angiotensin-converting enzyme (ACE) inhibitors and survival, SAVE (Survival and Ventricular Enlargement). Mortality curves in the SAVE study in patients with varying degrees of postinfarct ventricular dysfunction. In this study, 2231 patients with ejection fraction <40% were randomized to receive captopril (n=1115) or placebo (n=1116) 3–16 days after experiencing a transmural infarct. After 42 months, the captopril group (12.5–150 mg/day) had a significant reduction in overall mortality (-19%), number of reinfarctions(-25%), hospitalizations (-22%), and in the number of patients who developed clinical congestive heart failure. The mortality reduction appeared after 1 year of treatment. (From Pfeffer MA, et al. *N. Engl. J. Med.* 1992;**327**:669.)

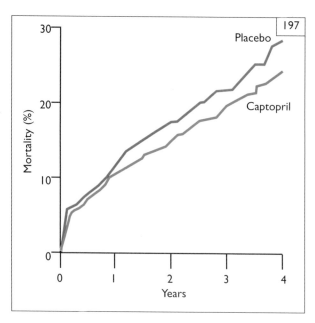

enjoyed a reduction in mortality of 27%. Zofenopril (SMILE Study) and trandolapril (TRACE Study) have similarly prolonged survival post-MI. In the SMILE Study, survival benefit was apparent after 3 months, and was further enhanced in patients with anterior MI (**198**). The TRACE Study reported an association between trandolapril and reduced sudden death. Meta-analysis of nearly 6000 participants of three post-MI studies further illustrated the benefits of ACE inhibitors in this setting (**199**).

Reduction of cardiovascular events
Analyses of data from the early ACE inhibitor-heart failure trials suggested that ACE inhibition in patients with low EFs reduced rates of subsequent MI. Suggested mechanisms included diminished progression of atherosclerosis, which might be promoted by an activated RAAS. The Heart Outcomes Prevention Evaluation (HOPE) Study investigated the impact of ACE inhibition with ramipril upon both cardiovascular mortality and events in over 9000

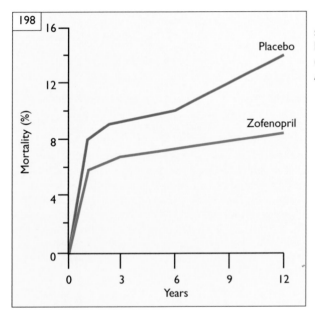

198 Angiotensin-converting enzyme inhibitors and survival after anterior myocardial infarction (MI). Patients were given zofenopril (n=772) or placebo (n=784) 24 hours post-MI for 6 weeks. (From Ambrosioni E, *et al. N. Engl. J. Med.* 1995;**332**:80.)

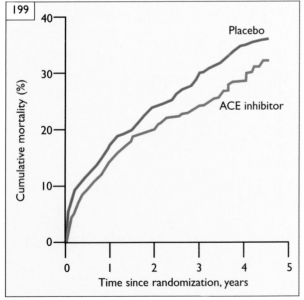

199 Meta-analysis of angiotensin-converting enzyme (ACE) inhibitors postmyocardial infarction in patients with left ventricular dysfunction (n=5966) in AIRE, SAVE and TRACE studies. Median follow-up was 31 months. Mortality was 23.4% for patients on ACE inhibitors versus 29% for patients on placebo (odds ratio 0.74, p<0.0001). (From Flather MD, *et al. Lancet* 2000;**355**:1575.) (For Trials see Appendix A.)

'high-risk' patients (i.e. with a previous vascular event, or with diabetes and one other cardiovascular risk factor, but no known HF). Treatment with ramipril reduced the rates of cardiovascular and all-cause deaths, as well as those for MI, stroke, worsening angina, and coronary revascularizations (**200**). Furthermore, treatment significantly reduced the rate of development of HF. Of note, the reduction in blood pressure in the ramipril group was small, and the observed benefits were independent of this reduction.

ADMINISTRATION OF ANGIOTENSON-CONVERTING ENZYME INHIBITORS

Initiation of ACE inhibitor treatment needs to be undertaken carefully as patients are often also taking diuretics, and the combination may lead to hypotension. However, it is no longer felt necessary to admit all patients into hospital in order to introduce these drugs, as was previously advocated. In certain patients (*Table 22*), treatment should still be commenced in a hospital setting. In others, the

200 Effect of ramipril in high-risk patients (HOPE study). Ramipril (n=651) reduces composite endpoint (death/myocardial infarction/cerebral vascular accident) compared with placebo (n=826) (14.1% versus 17.7%; risk ratio 0.78, p<0.001) at 4.5 year follow-up. The effect was independent of blood pressure reduction. (From Yusuf S, *et al. N. Engl. J. Med.* 2000;**342**:145.)

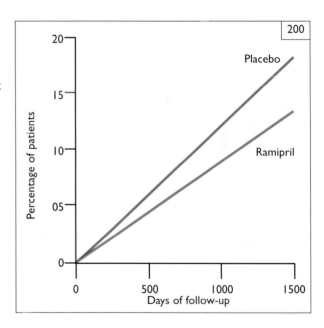

Table 22 Features necessitating hospitalization prior to starting angiotensin-converting enzyme inhibitors

◇ Severe heart failure

◇ Receiving high-dose diuretics or other vasodilators

◇ Hypotension (systolic BP <100 mmHg [13.3 kPa])

◇ Hypovolaemia

◇ Resting tachycardia

◇ Hyponatraemia (serum sodium <130 mmol/l [130 mEq/l])

BP: blood pressure.

dose of loop diuretic may need to be transiently reduced. Initial doses may cause hypotension and should be low, but subsequently need to be titrated upwards in order to achieve most benefit. For example, the Assessment of Treatment with Lisinopril and Survival (ATLAS) Trial, which studied outcome in patients with NYHA III HF, noted fewer hospitalizations for HF in those treated with relatively higher doses of lisinopril (2.5 mg versus 35 mg). There was no survival benefit with larger doses, however. Nevertheless, blockade of the RAAS is dose-related, and doses employed ought to be similar to those used in the relevant studies. Renal function should be monitored, especially in those likely to have renovascular disease. In particular, renal function in patients with bilateral renal artery stenosis is dependent on the RAAS, and ACE inhibition in these patients may lead to renal failure, and is contraindicated. ACE inhibitors are also contraindicated in pregnancy, and should also be avoided in patients with severe aortic stenosis, and in patients with a history of angio-oedema.

ETHNICITY AND ACE INHIBITION

The SOLVD studies included a significant proportion of black patients with LV dysfunction. Subanalysis of these data suggested that the black patients were at higher risk of death or hospitalization than their white counterparts, and also that their response to the ACE inhibitor, enalapril, was reduced. Previous studies have shown reduced hypertensive effect of ACE inhibitors in black people, and that plasma renin activity (a marker of activation of the RAAS) is lower in black people than in white people, suggesting that this system is less involved in the pathogenesis of hypertension and HF. Consequently, ACE inhibition is likely to be of less value in black patients. However, this remains controversial, and black patients should not be denied ACE inhibitors, as there is no superior alternative.

ADVERSE EFFECTS

In addition to causing first-dose hypotension, ACE inhibitors are frequently associated with a troublesome cough, an effect mediated by accumulation of bradykinin. This may remit with time or following dose reduction, but drug withdrawal may be necessary. The more specific angiotensin receptor blockers can be substituted in this scenario. The development of angio-oedema is also thought to be mediated by the bradykinin system. ACE inhibition may cause hyperkalaemia, and increased serum creatinine (although a rise of up to 15% is acceptable), and dose reduction or discontinuation may be necessary. ACE inhibitors may also cause an itchy, urticarial rash, which usually improves upon discontinuation.

Aldosterone escape

It is apparent that despite chronic ACE inhibitor treatment in patients with HF, angiotensin II and aldosterone may still be produced (aldosterone escape). This may be due, in part, to poor drug compliance, inadequate dose increases, or production from other pathways. For example, angiotensin II may also be generated by the action of the enzyme chymase upon angiotensin I, and aldosterone production may be stimulated by adrenocortico-trophic hormone. Persistently raised angiotensin II levels have been reported in between 15 and 50% of ACE-inhibited patients with HF, whereas aldosterone production is similarly sustained in up to 40%. The clinical sequelae of incomplete inhibition of the RAAS are unclear, although small studies have suggested associations with increased mortality and morbidity.

Thus, more effective attenuation of the RAAS may conceivably enhance treatment in a number of patients with HF. Drugs that block the angiotensin II receptors and aldosterone antagonists have been evaluated in the management of HF, and will be discussed further.

Angiotensin II receptor blockers

Angiotensin II receptor blockers (ARBs) block the action of angiotensin II at the type 1 receptor, which mediates hypertrophy. Their main role at present is in patients who are unable to tolerate ACE inhibitors due to cough or angio-oedema, an advantage of their more specific mode of action, which does not lead to accumulation of bradykinin. Whether they confer any mortality benefits in place of, or in addition to, ACE inhibitors is unclear at present, although further data are awaited.

The Symptom Tolerability Response to Exercise Trial of Candesartan in Heart failure (STRETCH) was conducted to study the effects of candesartan upon symptoms and exercise capacity in over 800 patients with HF. Following 12 weeks of treatment, candesartan was well tolerated, improved exercise performance and dyspnoea, and also reduced cardiothoracic ratio on chest X-ray. A systematic review of small trials (890 patients, NYHA II–III) comparing losartan to placebo suggested improved mortality with the ARB.

However, ARBs have not been shown to be superior to ACE inhibitors in treating HF. The

Evaluation of Losartan In The Elderly (ELITE) studies have compared losartan with captopril in treating HF. Although ELITE showed a trend towards reduced death and/or hospitalizations for HF with losartan, this study was designed to determine safety and efficacy, rather than survival. ELITE II, a larger study, showed no survival or hospitalization benefits of either drug, although losartan was tolerated better. Subsequently, the Valsartan Heart Failure Trial (Val-HeFT) assessed the value of valsartan as an adjunct to conventional HF therapies. Adjunctive valsartan was associated with a reduction in combined deaths/morbidity, largely driven by reduced hospitalizations for HF. The benefits, however, were most marked in those patients not taking ACE inhibitors, and, interestingly, the combination of ARB, ACE inhibitor and β-blocker was associated with increased mortality.

In 2003, more data on ARBs became available from the Candesartan in Heart failure Assessment of Reduction in Mortality and morbidity (CHARM) programme (**201, 202**), and the VALIANT

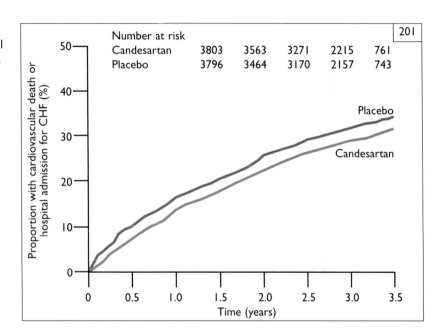

201 Effect of candesartan on cardiovascular mortality or hospital admission for chronic heart failure, the CHARM-Overall programme. Hazard ratio 0.84 (CI 0.77–0.91; p<0.0001). Adjusted hazard ratio 0.82, p<0.0001. (From Pfeffer MA, *et al. Lancet* 2003;**362**:759–766.)

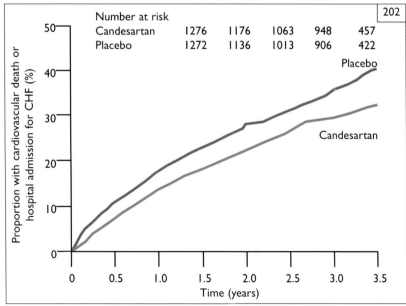

202 Effect of candesartan in patients with chronic heart failure (CHF) and reduced left ventricular systolic function taking angiotensin-converting enzyme inhibitors, CHARM-Added trial. Kaplan–Meier cumulative event curves are shown for primary outcome. Hazard ratio 0.85 (CI 0.75–0.96; p=0.011). Adjusted hazard ratio 0.85, p<0.01. (From McMurray JJV, *et al. Lancet* 2003;**362**:767–771.)

(Valsartan in Acute Myocardial Infarction Trial) trial (203). CHARM was specifically designed as three parallel, independent, integrated, randomized, double-blind, placebo-controlled clinical trials (CHARM-Added, CHARM-Alternative, CHARM-Preserved) comparing candesartan with placebo in three distinct but complementary populations of patients with symptomatic HF. In the CHARM-Overall combined analysis, 7599 patients with chronic HF were randomly assigned candesartan (n=3803, titrated to 32 mg once daily) or matching placebo (n=3796), and followed up for at least 2 years. After a median follow-up of 38 months, mortality was 23% in patients in the candesartan and 25% in the placebo group (adjusted hazard ratio (HR) 0.90). There were fewer cardiovascular deaths (18% vs. 20%, covariate adjusted HR 0.87) and hospital admissions for chronic HF (20% vs. 24%, p<0.0001) in the candesartan group. More patients discontinued candesartan than placebo because of concerns about renal function, hypotension, and hyperkalaemia, especially where candesartan was added to an ACE inhibitor (CHARM-Added, see below) or spironolactone.

In the CHARM-Added analysis, 2548 patients with NYHA functional class II–IV HF and LVEF ≤40%, and who were being treated with ACE inhibitors, were randomly assigned to candesartan (n=1276, target dose 32 mg once daily) or placebo (n=1272). After a median follow-up of 41 months, 38% of patients in the candesartan group and 42% in the placebo group experienced the primary outcome (unadjusted hazard ratio 0·85).

In the CHARM-Alternative analysis, 2028 patients with symptomatic HF and LVEF ≤40% who were not receiving ACE inhibitors because of previous intolerance, were randomly assigned candesartan (n=1013, target dose 32 mg once daily) or matching placebo (n=1015). The most common manifestation of ACE inhibitor intolerance was cough (72%), followed by symptomatic hypotension (13%) and renal dysfunction (12%). During a median follow-up of 33.7 months, 33% of the patients in the candesartan group and 40% in the placebo group had cardiovascular death or hospital admission for chronic HF (unadjusted HR 0.77). Study drug discontinuation rates were similar in the candesartan (30%) and placebo (29%) groups.

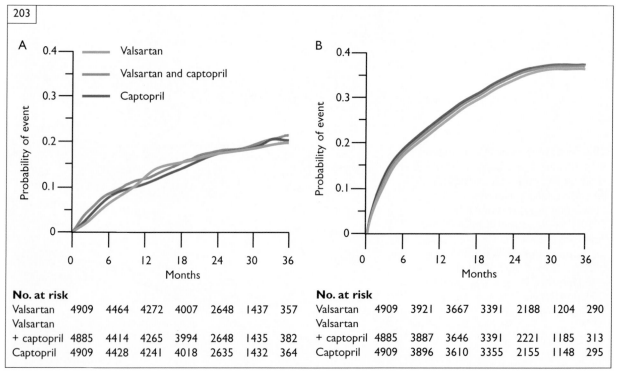

203 Kaplan–Meier estimates of the rate of death from any cause (A) and from cardiovascular causes, reinfarction, or hospitalization for heart failure (B) according to treatment group. For the rate of death from any cause, valsartan versus captopril p=0.98; valsartan-and-captopril versus captopril p=0.73. For the combined cardiovascular endpoints, valsartan versus captopril p=0.20; valsartan-and-captopril versus captopril p=0.37. (From Pfeffer MA, et al. N. Engl. J. Med. 2003; **349**:1893.)

The CHARM-Preserved analysis addressed the question of heart failure with preserved systolic function. The CHARM-Preserved randomly assigned 3023 patients to candesartan (n=1514, target dose 32 mg once daily) or matching placebo (n=1509). After a median follow-up of 36.6 months, 22% of the candesartan group and 24% of the placebo group experienced the primary outcome (unadjusted hazard ratio 0.89, p=0.118; covariate adjusted 0.86, p=0.051). Cardiovascular death did not differ between groups (170 vs. 170), but fewer patients in the candesartan group than in the placebo group were admitted to hospital for chronic HF (230 vs. 279, p=0.017). Thus, candesartan had some (modest) impact in preventing admissions for chronic HF among patients who have HF and preserved systolic function.

VALIANT was a double-blind trial, which compared the effect of the ARB valsartan, the ACE inhibitor captopril, and the combination of the two on mortality in patients with MI complicated by LV systolic dysfunction, HF, or both. Patients receiving conventional therapy were randomly assigned, 0.5–10 days after acute MI, to additional therapy with valsartan (4909 patients), valsartan plus captopril (4885 patients), or captopril (4909 patients). During a median follow-up of 24.7 months, 979 patients in the valsartan group died, as did 941 patients in the valsartan-and-captopril group and 958 patients in the captopril group (HR=1.0 for valsartan versus captopril; HR=0.98 for valsartan-and-captopril group versus captopril group). The valsartan-and-captopril group had the most drug-related adverse events. Thus, valsartan was as effective as captopril in patients who are at high risk for cardiovascular events after MI. Unfortunately, combining valsartan with captopril increased the rate of adverse events without improving survival.

Aldosterone antagonists

The aldosterone antagonist spironolactone (also known as aldactone) has been used for many years in the treatment of hyperaldosteronism, either in primary form (Conn's syndrome), or when resulting from hepatic cirrhosis, where it is used to reduce ascites. Aldosterone has deleterious effects upon the heart and vasculature (**204**), which may be alleviated by spironolactone.

204 Mechanism of action of aldosterone inhibitors. The beneficial effects of spironolactone derive from the direct and competitive blockade of specific aldosterone receptors. Aldosterone inhibitors therefore have three types of effects: (1) diuretic effect, which is most noticeable when fluid retention and increased levels of aldosterone are present; (2) antiarrhythmic effect, mediated by the correction of hypokalaemia and hypomagnesaemia; (3) antifibrotic effect (demonstrated in animal models) which can contribute to a decrease in the progression of structural changes in patients with heart failure.

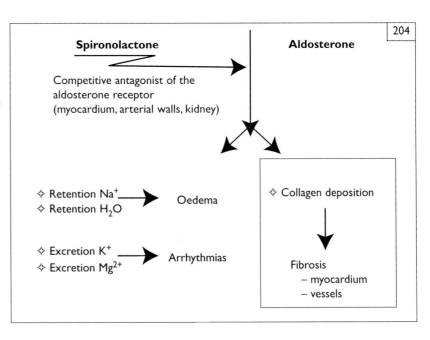

The Randomized ALdactone Evaluation Study (RALES) assessed the efficacy of spironolactone in treating severe HF when added to ACE inhibitors, loop diuretics and, in some patients, digoxin. The addition of spironolactone was associated with marked reductions in mortality and hospitalizations, with recipients also noting symptom improvement. Significant hyperkalaemia was not apparent with spironolactone treatment in this trial, although gynaecomastia/breast pain occurred in 10% of men. The results of this trial prompted widespread use of spironolactone in severe HF, particularly in patients not able to tolerate β-blockers.

More recently, epleronone, a more specific aldosterone antagonist has been evaluated in the treatment of systolic HF following MI in the Epleronone Post-Acute Myocardial Infarction Heart Failure Efficacy and Survival Study (EPHESUS). Over 6500 patients were randomized to either epleronone or placebo in addition to conventional treatment post-MI. Epleronone in addition to ACE inhibitors/ARB and β-blockade was associated with a reduction in all-cause (relative risk= 0.85) and cardiac mortality, sudden death, and the combined endpoint of cardiac deaths/hospitalizations (relative risk= 0.87). The incidence of serious hyperkalaemia was increased in the study group, although the rate of serious hypokalaemia was decreased.

Diuretics

Diuretics are used as the first-line drug agents in HF (*Table 23*). The first diuretics, which were organic mercurial compounds, were introduced in the 1920s, with thiazides following in the 1950s. Diuretics have long been recognized to confer symptomatic improvement in acute and chronic HF, and their use is associated with favourable effects upon haemodynamics and exercise capacity. However, unlike ACE inhibitors and β-adrenoceptor blockers, there have been no large, randomized control studies that have revealed diuretic-related survival benefit.

LOOP DIURETICS

The loop diuretics (frusemide [furosemide], bumetanide [bumetadine], torasemide [torsemide], and ethacrynic acid) are so-named because of their site of action (205) at the ascending limb of the loop of Henle within the nephron. Upon their secretion into the tubular fluid by proximal tubular cells, they block the reabsorption of sodium, chloride, and water (at the Na^+–K^+–H_2O co-transporter), resulting in the excretion of 20–25% of the total filtered sodium load, and a potent diuresis. Their onset of action is rapid, and the half-lives range from 1 to 4 hours, allowing twice daily administration. Higher doses may be required in renal impairment, when the glomerular filtration rate (GFR) falls below 25 ml/minute. Additionally, intravenous use is associated with transient venodilatation, which is particularly beneficial in acute HF. This effect may be mediated by

Table 23 Diuretics (oral) dosages and side-effects

Drug	Initial dose (mg)		Maximum recommended daily dose (mg)	
Loop diuretics				
Bumetanide	0.5–1.0		5–10	
Frusemide	20–40		250–500	
Torasemide	5–10		100–200	
Thiazides*				
Bendroflumethiazide (previously bendrofluazide)	2.5		5	
Indapamide	2.5		2.5	
Metolazone	2.5		10	
Potassium-sparing diuretics	+ACEI	-ACEI	+ACEI	-ACEI
Amiloride	2.5	5	20	40
Triamterene	25	50	100	200
Spironolactone see *Table 24*				

ACEI: angiotensin-converting enzyme inhibitor.
* May be effective when added to loop diuretics when fluid retention is resistant, but can promote dramatic diuresis and disturbance in fluid balance and electrolytes. Patient must be closely monitored and specialist advice is required.

prostaglandins, and has been reported to be attenuated by nonsteroidal anti-inflammatory drugs (NSAIDs) and aspirin.

Frusemide and bumetanide are the most common loop diuretics used. The oral absorption of bumetanide exceeds that of frusemide. Frusemide is excreted renally, whereas bumetanide and torasemide undergo hepatic degradation. Thus, in patients with renal dysfunction, the plasma half-life of frusemide is increased. In contrast, the half-lives of bumetanide and torasemide are unaffected by renal impairment, but are increased in patients with hepatic impairment.

Comparisons of survival of patients with HF related to frusemide and torasemide have suggested benefit with the latter agent. For example, the TORIC study analyzed survival in patients with HF (NYHA II–III) followed up for 9 months. Torasemide use was associated with a reduction in total and cardiac deaths, with more stable control of serum potassium apparent. However, this trial was not blinded, and was not originally designed to assess mortality. Moreover, the concomitant use of ACE inhibitors and β-blockers was low.

THIAZIDE DIURETICS

Thiazide diuretics (e.g. bendroflumethiazide and hydrochlorothiazide) and thiazide-related diuretics (e.g. chlorthalidone) are commonly used in the treatment of hypertension, and may also be used to treat HF. They prevent sodium reabsorption in the early segment of the distal tubule (205), although their diuretic effect is up to eight times less potent than loop diuretics, and they are less effective when GFR <30 ml/minute. Thus, these drugs are more useful in the treatment of milder degrees of HF. They act within 2 hours of oral administration, and have longer half-lives than loop diuretics. Adjunctive use with loop diuretics results in a more comprehensive nephron blockade, and a marked diuresis which is beneficial when higher doses of loop diuretics are ineffective alone. The thiazide-like drug metolazone is particularly potent in combination treatment, and must be used cautiously, with electrolyte monitoring.

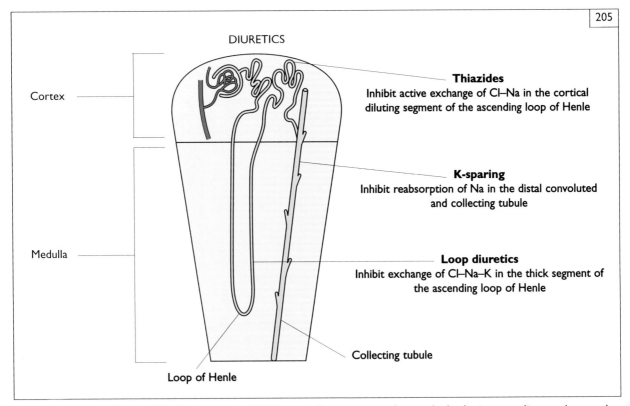

205 Classification and mechanisms of action of diuretics. Diuretics are drugs which eliminate sodium and water by acting directly on the kidney. The diuretics are the primary line of therapy for the majority of patients with heart failure and pulmonary congestion. Diuretics (loop, thiazides, and potassium-sparing) produce a net loss of sodium and water, decreasing acute symptoms which result from fluid retention (dyspnoea, oedema).

POTASSIUM-SPARING DIURETICS

This group of diuretics includes amiloride, triamterene, and spironolactone (*Tables 23, 24*). These agents block the luminal Na^+ channels in the distal nephron, although they are relatively weak diuretics in themselves, with only 5% of filtered sodium excreted.

Table 24 Practical recommendations for the use of spironolactone

Which dose of spironolactone?

Dose (mg)

12.5–25 daily

◇ 50 mg may be advised by a specialist if heart failure deteriorates and no problem with hyperkalaemia

How to use

◇ Start at 25 mg OD
◇ Check blood chemistry at 1, 4, 8, and 12 weeks; 6, 9, and 12 months; 6 monthly thereafter
◇ If K^+ rises to between 5.5 and 5.9 mmol/l (mEq/l) or creatinine rises to 200 µmol/l (2.3 mg/dl), reduce dose to 25 mg on alternate days and monitor blood chemistry closely
◇ If K^+ rises to ≥6.0 mmol/l (mEq/l) or creatinine to >200 µmol/l (2.3 mg/dl), stop spironolactone and seek specialist advice

Advice to patient

◇ Explain expected benefits
◇ Treatment is given to improve symptoms, to prevent worsening of heart failure, and to increase survival
◇ Symptoms improve within a few weeks to a few months of starting treatment
◇ Avoid NSAIDs not prescribed by a physician (self-purchased 'over the counter' treatment [e.g. ibuprofen])
◇ Temporarily stop spironolactone if diarrhoea and/or vomiting occurs and contact physician

Problem solving

Worsening renal function/hyperkalaemia

◇ See 'How to use'
◇ Major concern is hyperkalaemia (≥6.0 mmol/l [mEq/l]) though this was uncommon in the RALES clinical trial; a K^+ level at the higher end of normal range may be desirable in patients with heart failure, particularly if taking digoxin
◇ Some 'low salt' substitutes have a high K^+ content
◇ Male patients may develop breast discomfort and/or gynaecomastia. NSAID: nonsteroidal anti-inflammatory drugs. (From McMurray JJV, et al. Eur. J. Heart Fail. 2001;**3**:495–502.)

They are mainly used to prevent hypokalaemia, which may result from use of loop or thiazide diuretics. Several potassium-sparing diuretics have been combined with either loop or thiazide agents, and this may result in improved compliance, particularly among elderly patients. Spironolactone, an antagonist of aldosterone, improves survival in moderate to severe HF when used with diuretics, ACE inhibitors, and β-blockers (see above).

ADVERSE EFFECTS

Diuretic use is associated with many metabolic abnormalities which necessitate careful use. Hyponatraemia and hypokalaemia are common, and loop or thiazide agents are often used with potassium supplements or in combination with agents such as amiloride. However, such supplements should not be used with ACE inhibitors due to the risk of hyperkalaemia. Loop and thiazide agents may be associated with hypocalcaemia and hypercalcaemia, respectively, and both groups increase serum urate, increasing the risk of developing gout. Large, intravenous doses of loop diuretics may be ototoxic, and intravenous bumetanide administration has been reported to cause severe myalgia. Finally, excessive doses, especially when used with ACE inhibitors, can cause hypovolaemia and result in uraemia and, if uncorrected, renal failure.

DIURETIC RESISTANCE

Following initiation of diuretic therapy, sodium and water loss results in symptom improvement and weight loss. However, inbetween doses, sodium loss is attenuated in order to prevent depletion of body stores, and a rebound period of sodium reabsorption follows. The prevention of resolution of oedema by this homeostatic mechanism is characteristic of diuretic resistance, and this phenomenon may lengthen the duration of hospital admissions with HF. Underlying mechanisms include sodium retention, due to activation of the RAAS or due to a compensatory increase in reabsorption in the distal nephron; renal dysfunction, with decreased tubular drug delivery; and altered diuretic bioavailability, resulting from diminished oral absorption in decompensated patients.

Strategies to overcome diuretic resistance (*Table 25*) include ensuring dietary sodium is restricted, and NSAIDs are avoided due to their negative effect upon renal perfusion. Indeed, an exaggerated contraction in circulating volume (especially with concurrent use) may exacerbate the reduction in renal perfusion, and further diminish diuretic effect. Although increasing doses of oral loop diuretics may alleviate some resistance, the addition of a thiazide diuretic is frequently beneficial. Furthermore, in severe cases, intravenous administration of loop diuretics is often required, possibly overcoming problems with intestinal absorption. Continuous intravenous infusion may be superior to bolus administration, perhaps by overcoming the rebound increase in sodium reabsorption associated with the intervals between doses. This results in a more rapid diuresis and weight loss, with shorter hospital stays resulting.

Further reading

CONSENSUS Trial Study Group. Effects of enalapril on mortality in severe congestive heart failure: results of the Cooperative North Scandinavian Enalapril Survival Study. *N. Engl. J. Med.* 1987;**316**:1429–1435.

DeBruyne LK. Mechanisms and management of diuretic resistance in congestive heart failure. *Postgrad. Med. J.* 2003;**79**(931):268–271.

Epleronone Post-Acute Myocardial Infarction Heart Failure Efficacy and Survival Study (EPHESUS) Investigators. *N. Engl. J. Med.* 2003;**348**:1309–1321.

Granger CB, McMurray JJV, Yusuf S, *et al.* for the CHARM Investigators and Committees. Effects of candesartan in patients with chronic heart failure and reduced left ventricular systolic function intolerant to angiotensin-converting enzyme inhibitors: the CHARM-Alternative trial. *Lancet* 2003;**362**:772–776.

Heart Outcomes Prevention Evaluation (HOPE) Study Investigators. Effects of an angiotensin converting enzyme inhibitor, ramipril, on cardiovascular events in high-risk patients. *N. Engl. J. Med.* 2000;**342**:145–153.

McMurray JJV, Östergren J, Swedberg K, *et al.* for the CHARM Investigators and Committees. Effects of candesartan in patients with chronic heart failure and reduced left ventricular systolic function taking angiotensin-converting enzyme inhibitors: the CHARM-Added trial. *Lancet* 2003;**362**:767–771.

Pfeffer MA, Braunwald E, Moyé LA, *et al.* Effect of captopril on mortality and morbidity in patients with left ventricular dysfunction after myocardial infarction: results of the Survival and Ventricular Enlargement Trial. *N. Engl. J. Med.* 1992;**327**:669–677.

Pfeffer MA, Swedberg K, Granger CB, *et al.* for the CHARM Investigators and Committees. Effects of candesartan on mortality and morbidity in patients with chronic heart failure: the CHARM-Overall programme. *Lancet* 2003;**362**:759–766.

Randomized Aldactone Evaluation Study (RALES) Investigators. The effect of spironolactone on morbidity and mortality in patients with severe heart failure. *N. Engl. J. Med.* 1999;**341**:709–717.

Yusuf S, Pfeffer MA, Swedberg K, *et al.* for the CHARM Investigators and Committees. Effects of candesartan in patients with chronic heart failure and preserved left ventricular ejection fraction: the CHARM-Preserved Trial. *Lancet* 2003;**362**:777–778.

Table 25 Strategies to overcome diuretic resistance (increasing weight/peripheral oedema despite adequate doses of loop diuretic)

- Ensure low sodium diet
- Restrict fluids to <2 l/day
- Increase dose of loop diuretic
- Consider a short course of additional thiazide (such as metolazone 5 mg/OD × 3 days)
- Consider changing frusemide (furosemide) to bumetanide (1 mg bumetanide for each 40 mg frusemide)
- Consider IV bolus frusemide (change oral dose to the same dose IV, in two divided doses)
- Consider IV infusion frusemide (one strategy is to give half daily dose as a bolus at 8 am then the remaining frusemide as a continuous infusion over 8 hours)

Chapter six

Beta-blockers and inotropes

Beta-blockers

β-adrenoceptor blockers have been used as cardiovascular drugs for decades now, having been discovered in the 1950s. They have a well-established role in the management of ischaemic heart disease, arrhythmias, and hypertension (*Table 26*). β-blockers reduce heart rate and contractility, thereby reducing myocardial oxygen demand; the reduction in heart rate allows for increased coronary flow during diastole, which improves oxygen supply. Therefore, β-blockers are useful in treating ischaemic heart disease. Furthermore, certain β-blockers have been shown to reduce mortality and recurrent ischaemia after myocardial infarction (MI). β-blockers are thought to reduce blood pressure via a central action, in part, possibly augmenting the effects of reduced cardiac output.

β-blockade would appear a logical therapy in heart failure (HF), given the characteristic chronic activation of the sympathetic system among sufferers of this condition. However, β-blockers were previously avoided in patients with HF, because of fears of exacerbations related to their negative inotropic effect. Subsequently, several randomized, controlled clinical trials have shown favourable mortality and morbidity outcomes resulting from the use of β-blockers in all grades of HF.

MECHANISMS OF ACTION

β-blockers exert a negatively inotropic effect upon normal myocardium, yet improve function in failing myocardium. A persistent hyperadrenergic state is central to the development of HF, but any improved contractility that one might expect is negated by myocardial insensitivity to adrenergic stimulation. Myocardial β_1 adrenoceptor density was shown to be reduced in patients with HF in the early 1980s, but was shown to be increased by β-blockade. Furthermore, excessive sympathetic stimulation may

induce myocyte apoptosis, which may be ameliorated by β-blockade. Additional mechanisms may include promoting more favourable calcium loading within myocytes or altered gene expression.

STUDIES OF BETA-BLOCKERS IN HEART FAILURE

Early, uncontrolled studies of β-blockade in patients with symptomatic congestive cardiomyopathy were conducted in the 1970s, and reported clinical and haemodynamic improvement, although β-blockers were still widely regarded as harmful in HF at this time. In the β-blockers in Heart Attack Trial (BHAT), propranolol given after MI was particularly beneficial in those with worse left ventricular function prior to treatment (**206**). Subsequently, in

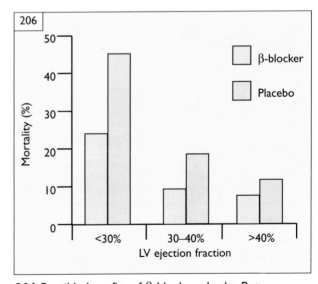

206 Possible benefits of β-blockers. In the Beta-Blockers in Heart Attack Trial (BHAT), the decrease in mortality associated with propranolol use was found to be inversely related to the pretreatment ejection fraction. LV: left ventricular. (From BHAT. *J. Am. Med. Assoc.* 1982;**247**:1704–1714.)

Table 26 Practical recommendations on the use of beta-blockers

Which β-blocker and what dose?
Only two β-blockers are licensed for the treatment of heart failure in the UK at the time of issue of this guideline.

	Starting dose (mg)	Target dose (mg)
Bisoprolol	1.25 OD	10 OD
Carvedilol	3.125 BID	25–50 BID*

* Carvedilol maximum dose 25 mg BID if severe heart failure. For patients with mild to moderate heart failure, maximum dose 50 mg BID if weight >85 kg (190 lb), otherwise maximum dose 25 mg BID.

Metoprolol is not licensed for heart failure in the UK; however, in, for example, Australia, India, The Netherlands, and the USA, it is indicated for heart failure.

	Starting dose (mg)	Maximum daily dose (mg)
Metoprolol tartrate	5 BID*	50 BID*
Metoprolol succinate	25 OD**	200 OD**

* Doses used in the COMET trial   ** Doses used in the MERIT-HF trial

How to use
✧ Start with a low dose (see above)
✧ Double dose at not less than 2 weekly intervals
✧ Aim for target dose (see above) or, failing that, the highest tolerated dose
✧ Remember some β-blocker is better than none
✧ Monitor heart rate, BP, clinical status (symptoms, signs especially signs of congestion, body weight)
✧ Check blood electrolytes, urea, creatinine 1–2 weeks after initiation and 1–2 weeks after final dose titration
✧ When to down-titrate/stop up-titration see 'Problem solving'

Advice to patient
✧ Explain expected benefits
✧ Emphasize that treatment is given as much to prevent worsening heart failure as to improve symptoms; β-blockers also increase survival
✧ If symptom improvement occurs, this may develop slowly (3–6 months or longer)
✧ Temporary symptomatic deterioration may occur (estimated 20–30% of cases) during initiation/up-titration phase
✧ Advise patient to report deterioration (see 'Problem solving') and that deterioration (tiredness, fatigue, breathlessness) can usually be easily managed by adjustment of other medication; patients should be advised not to stop β-blocker therapy without consulting their physician
✧ Patients should be encouraged to weigh themselves daily (after waking, before dressing, after voiding, before eating) and to consult their physician if they have persistent weight gain

Problem solving
Worsening symptoms/signs (e.g. increasing dyspnoea, fatigue, oedema, weight gain)
✧ If increasing congestion, double the dose of diuretic and/or halve dose of β-blocker (if increasing diuretic has no effect)
✧ If marked fatigue (and/or bradycardia, see below) halve the dose of β-blocker (rarely necessary)
✧ Review patient in 1–2 weeks; if not improved seek specialist advice
✧ If serious deterioration, halve the dose of β-blocker or stop this treatment (rarely necessary) and seek specialist advice
Low heart rate
✧ If <50 bpm and worsening symptoms, halve dose of β-blocker or, if severe deterioration, stop β-blocker (rarely necessary)
✧ Consider the need to continue other medication with drugs that slow the heart (e.g. digoxin, amiodarone, diltiazem) and discontinue if possible
✧ Arrange ECG to exclude heart block
✧ Seek specialist advice
Asymptomatic low blood pressure
✧ Does not usually require any change in therapy
Symptomatic hypotension
✧ If low BP causes dizziness, light-headedness, or confusion consider discontinuing drugs such as nitrates, calcium channel blockers, and other vasodilators
✧ If no signs/symptoms of congestion, consider reducing diuretic dose
✧ If these measures do not solve the problem seek specialist advice

NB: β-blockers should not be stopped suddenly unless absolutely necessary (there is a risk of rebound increase in myocardial ischaemia/infarction and arrhythmia). Ideally, specialist advice should be sought before treatment is discontinued. BP: blood pressure; ECG: electrocardiogram. (From McMurray JJV, et al. Eur. J. Heart Fail. 2001;**3**:495–502.)

the early 1990s, the Metoprolol in Dilated Cardiomyopathy (MDC) study reported functional and quality of life improvement associated with metoprolol therapy. Retrospective analysis of data from the Survival and Ventricular Enlargement (SAVE) trial, which evaluated the effect of the angiotensin-converting enzyme (ACE) inhibitor

enalapril on survival post-MI, noted improved survival among patients also receiving β-blockers (*Table 27*).

Large prospective randomized survival studies have since been conducted, and the majority have revealed significant survival and symptomatic benefit in adding β-blockers to ACE inhibitors (*Table 28*).

The US Carvedilol Study assessed outcome of treatment with carvedilol in patients with predominantly mild–moderate HF. This study amalgamated results from four separate trials, with a total of 1094 patients recruited. Carvedilol treatment was asssociated with significantly improved mortality and hospitalization rates, although mortality was not a primary end point. Two other agents, bisoprolol and metoprolol, were evaluated in the second Cardiac Insufficiency Bisoprolol Study (CIBIS II) and Metoprolol Controlled Release/Extended Release Randomized Intervention Trial (MERIT-HF), respectively. These studies reported similar reductions in both mortality and hospitalizations in patients with moderate-severe (CIBIS II) and mild–moderate (MERIT-HF) severity. Analysis of metoprolol therapy in patients with severe (NYHA IV) HF revealed

Table 27 Mortality of patients on beta-blockers with angiotensin-converting enzyme inhibitors (n=2231)

		β-blocker	
		Yes (%)	No (%)
ACE inhibitor	Yes (%)	13.3	24.3
	No (%)	19.5	27.7

Patients were postmyocardial infarction with ejection fraction <40%. At median follow-up of 42 months mortality was lower in patients on β-blockers, regardless of randomization to placebo or angiotenson-converting enzyme (ACE) inhibitor therapy. Mortality was lowest when β-blockers were combined with ACE inhibitors and was maximal when neither drug was used. (From SAVE. *Circulation* 1995;**92**:3132.)

Table 28 Major studies showing benefits of beta-blockers in heart failure

Study	Year	Drug	n	NYHA Class	Mortality reduction (%)	Hospitalizations reduction (%)
US Carvedilol	1996	Carvedilol	1094	II–III	65	27
CIBIS-II	1999	Bisoprolol	2647	III–IV	34	20
MERIT-HF	1999	Metoprolol	3991	II–III	34	18
COPERNICUS	2001	Carvedilol	2289	IV	35	20

(From Gheorghiade M, *et al. Circulation* 2003;**107**:1570.)

Table 29 Effect of metoprolol and placebo treatment on survival and hospitalization risk in class III and IV heart failure

Endpoint	Metoprolol (n)	Placebo (n)	Risk reduction (%)	p value
Total mortality	45	72	39	0.0086
Cardiovascular mortality	40	70	44	0.0028
Sudden death	22	39	45	0.024
Death from worsening heart failure	13	28	55	0.015
Total hospitalizations	273	363	27	0.0037
Total hospitalizations due to worsening heart failure	105	187	45	<0.0001

(From Goldstein S, *et al. J. Am. Coll. Cardiol.* 2001;**38**:932–938.)

particular benefit in this group (*Tables 29, 30*). Carvedilol was assessed again, in patients with severe HF and left ventricular ejection fraction (LVEF) <25%, in the Carvedilol Prospective Randomized Cumulative Survival (COPERNICUS) study. Significant mortality and morbidity benefits were again apparent.

It should not be assumed that all β-blockers will improve clinical outcomes. In particular, treatment with bucindolol, an agent with intrinsic sympathomimetic activity and vasodilating properties, was not associated with mortality reduction in patients with moderate–severe HF in the Beta-blocker Evaluation Survival Trial (BEST).

CHOICE OF BETA-BLOCKER

β-blockers have varying pharmacological properties, which may be advantageous in different situations. For example, metoprolol and bisoprolol are examples of cardioselective β-blockers, and block β_1 adrenoceptors relatively better than the β_2 subtype. These drugs have a less marked effect on airways obstruction than nonselective agents. Carvedilol is a nonselective agent, which also blocks α_1 receptors, thus conferring vasodilatory capacity. This may be of benefit for patients with peripheral vascular disease.

At present, it is unclear as to which of the proven β-blockers (bisoprolol, metoprolol, or carvedilol) is superior. The Carvedilol or Metoprolol European

Trial (COMET) has recently addressed this issue: over 3000 patients were randomized to either metoprolol or carvedilol, with mortality significantly lower with carvedilol (**207**). COMET was a multicentre, double-blind, and randomized parallel group trial, which assigned 1511 patients with chronic HF to treatment with carvedilol (target dose 25 mg twice daily) and 1518 to metoprolol (metoprolol tartrate, target dose 50 mg twice daily). After a mean study duration of 58 months, the all-cause mortality was 34% for carvedilol and 40% for metoprolol (hazard ratio, HR 0.83, p=0.0017). The composite endpoint of mortality or all-cause

Table 30 Comparison of findings in subanalysis and entire MERIT heart failure (HF) cohort

Endpoint	Reductions in entire MERIT-HF cohort (%)	Reductions in class III/I MERIT-HF subset (%)
Total mortality	-34	-39
Sudden death	-41	-45
Death due to worsening HF	-49	-55

(From Goldstein S, et al. J. Am. Coll. Cardiol. 2001;**38**:932–938.)

207 Carvedilol versus metoprolol in patients with chronic heart failure (the Carvedilol Or Metoprolol European Trial (COMET). (From Poole-Wilson PA, et al. Lancet 2003;**362**:7–13.)

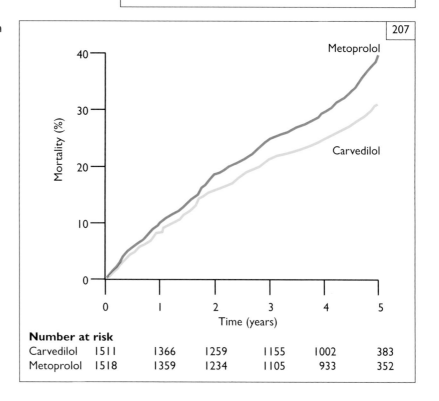

Number at risk						
Carvedilol	1511	1366	1259	1155	1002	383
Metoprolol	1518	1359	1234	1105	933	352

86

admission occurred in 1116 (74%) of 1511 on carvedilol and in 1160 (76%) of 1518 on metoprolol (HR 0.94, p=0.122). While COMET suggests that carvedilol extended survival compared with metoprolol, it is of note that the formulation of metoprolol used in this trial differed from the controlled/extended release formulation used in MERIT-HF. Modified release metoprolol, at present, is unlicensed for use in HF in the UK, whereas bisoprolol has not been approved for similar use in the US.

ADMINISTRATION

Patients with HF require careful assessment prior to, and after, initiation of β-blocker therapy. Contraindications to use include clinically unstable HF (evidenced by increases in body weight or diuretic dose, worsening of HF symptoms, need for intravenous diuretics or inotropes), evidence of reversible airways disease, hypotension (systolic blood pressure <85 mmHg [11.3 kPa]), or high-grade atrioventricular block.

β-blockade may still cause worsening of symptoms, so initial doses used are small; patients should be warned of potential symptoms suggesting deterioration. Such deterioration may be transient, but in some cases, withdrawal is necessary. Patients should be told that symptoms might not improve until a few weeks after commencing treatment. Regular clinical reviews should be undertaken in order to increase doses safely to the targets used in trials (*Table 31*). Specialized HF clinics may be of value in dose titration, amongst other roles.

Data have shown that those patients unable to tolerate the maximum doses of β-blocker (typically the elderly or those with most severe HF) will still benefit from submaximal doses. For example, a subgroup analysis of CIBIS II revealed significant reductions in all-cause mortality in those treated with bisoprolol, which were irrespective of the dose reached. Furthermore, discontinuing bisoprolol treatment was associated with increased mortality (relative hazard 2.13, p=0.0002). β-blockers, of course, are adjuncts to treatment with ACE inhibitors (and digoxin), but can be commenced even when ACE inhibitor titration is submaximal.

Positive inotropes

Positive inotropes are classified according to mechanism of action (*Table 32*). This section will discuss the effects of the cardiac glycosides (digoxin), sympathomimetics, and phosphodiesterase inhibitors. A novel agent, levosimendan, will also be considered.

Table 31 Beta-blocker dose titration			
	Bisoprolol	**Carvedilol**	**Metoprolol CR/XL**
Start	1.25 mg OD	3.125 mg BID	12.5 mg/25 mg OD*
Wk 1	2.5 mg OD		
Wk 2	3.75 mg OD	6.25 mg BID	25 mg/50 mg OD
Wk 3	5 mg OD		
Wk 4		12.5 mg BID	50 mg/100mg OD
Wk 6		25mg BID (MAX)	100 mg/200mg OD
Wk 7	7.5mg OD		
Wk 8			200 mg OD (MAX)
Wk 11	10 mg OD (MAX)		

*In MERIT-HF, patients in NYHA III–IV initially received 12.5 mg OD; those in NYHA II were started on 25 mg OD.
MERIT-HF: Metoprolol CR/XL Randomized Intervention Trial in Congestive Heart Failure; NYHA: New York Heart Association.

Table 32 Positive inotropes

Cardiac glycosides

Sympathomimetics

✧ Catecholamines

✧ β-adrenergic agonists

Phosphodiesterase inhibitors

✧ Amrinone

✧ Enoximone

✧ Milrinone

✧ Piroximone

Others

The use of inotropic agents in heart failure is intended to increase contractility and cardiac output. Theoretically, their use should be greatest in heart failure associated with a decrease in systolic function and marked cardiomegaly, depression of ejection fraction, and elevated left ventricular filling pressure. In addition to the cardiac glycosides, other positive inotropic agents include: (a) the sympathomimetics, represented by the β1 agonists (which stimulate cardiac contractility) and β2-adrenergics (vasodilators). Both groups increase the intracellular concentration of cAMP by stimulating the activity of adenylate cyclase which converts ATP to cAMP; (b) phosphodiesterase inhibitors, which inhibit the enzyme that breaks down cAMP, increase cardiac contractility and have arteriovenous vasodilatory effect; (c) other inotropic drugs including glucagon and Na^+ channel agonists.

DIGOXIN

The cardiac glycoside digoxin has been used in the treatment of HF since 1785, when William Withering of Birmingham published an account of the benefits of digitalis in treating 'dropsy'. Digoxin is extracted from the leaves of the plant *Digitalis purpurea* (the foxglove). Indeed, the foxglove is believed to have been used for medicinal reasons in Ancient Rome. Currently, there is wide variation in the use of digoxin in HF. In the UK, its main role is in patients who have HF with associated atrial fibrillation (AF), where it is valuable in reducing uncontrolled ventricular rates. In the US, digoxin is routinely used in the treatment of HF due to left ventricular systolic dysfunction, even in patients who remain in sinus rhythm.

Mechanism of action

The inotropic effect of the cardiac glycosides is mediated by their inhibition of the Na-K ATPase pump (**208**). This pump is found in a variety of tissues including human myocardium, and is responsible for the active transport of sodium and potassium across cell membranes. Inhibition by drugs such as digoxin causes a rise in intracellular sodium, which, in turn, permits net calcium influx via the Na-Ca exchanger. Calcium, upon incorporation into the contractile apparatus, augments contractility. Cardiac glycosides also reduce conduction within the atrioventricular node, which reduces ventricular rates in patients with persistent AF.

208 Mechanism of action of digoxin. Digoxin attaches to specific receptors which form a part of the enzyme, Na^+/K^+-dependent ATP-ase (sodium pump), inhibiting it. This blockade produces a progressive increase in the intracellular concentration of sodium, which in turn activates the exchange of Na^+-Ca^{++} and increases the influx of Ca^{++} and its intracellular concentration, $[Ca^{++}]i$. This increase in the $[Ca^{++}]i$ at the level of the contractile proteins explains the resultant increase in cardiac contractility.

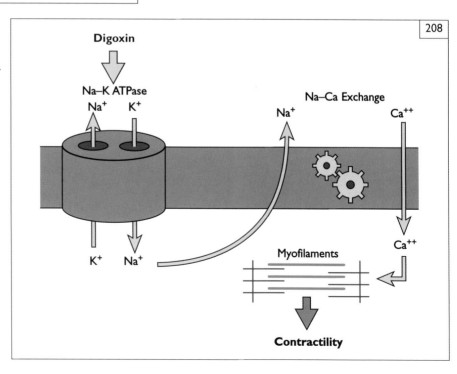

Digoxin and heart failure
Digoxin use is associated with improved symptoms and functional capacity, with reduced hospitalizations for HF. Studies which have assessed the effects of digoxin withdrawal have noted adverse outcomes after discontinuation. For example, the Randomised Assessment of Digoxin and Inhibitors of Angiotensin-converting Enzyme (RADIANCE) study recruited 178 patients with LVEF <35% and NYHA I–III. Digoxin withdrawal was associated with significant worsening of HF, and significant decreases in exercise and LVEF (**209**). Retrospective analysis revealed that the benefits of continuing digoxin were unrelated to serum digoxin levels.

The effect of digoxin upon mortality was studied in the Digitalis Investigation Group (DIG) trial. In the trial 6800 subjects in sinus rhythm with HF due to systolic dysfunction (and receiving diuretics and ACE inhibitors) were randomized to digoxin or placebo. Overall, there were no differences in mortality between the two groups; a reduction in death due to worsening HF was countered by an increase in deaths from other causes (**210**). The digoxin group did, however, benefit from significantly fewer hospitalizations for worsening HF. Post-hoc analyses of this study have revealed that women treated with digoxin encountered higher mortality rates compared to women treated with placebo, although the mechanisms for this association are unclear. In men, those with relatively lower digoxin levels experienced lower rates of (all-cause) mortality.

Digoxin should be used for symptom relief in patients whose symptoms are refractory to treatment with diuretics, ACE inhibitors, and β-blockers, particularly those with a persistent tachycardia or third heart sound.

Administration
Rapid digoxin loading is mainly required in the context of controlling rapid ventricular rates in AF. In HF, typical initial doses of 125–250 µg twice daily for 5 days, with subsequent reduction, will usually suffice. Digoxin has a narrow therapeutic index, and plasma levels should be within the range of 0.5–2.0 ng/ml. Digoxin has a long plasma half-life (36 hours), and undergoes renal excretion. Therefore, particular care must be used in treating the elderly and those with renal impairment. Certain drugs (e.g. amiodarone) may also increase plasma digoxin levels. The pharmokinetics of digoxin are summarized in *Table 33*.

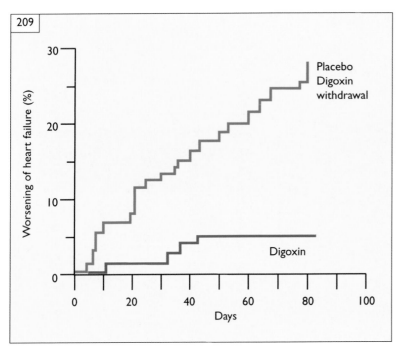

209 Effect of digoxin on morbidity. The RADIANCE trial analyzed clinical evolution in 178 patients with heart failure of functional classes II–III and left ventricular ejection fraction (LVEF) <35% treated with digoxin and diuretics and angiotensin-converting enzyme inhibitors (ACEI). Patients either continued their dose of digoxin between 0.125 and 0.5 mg/day with serum levels of 0.7–2.0 ng/ml (n=85), or discontinued digoxin and received placebo instead (n=93). After 100 days of treatment, digoxin withdrawal produced a significant worsening in heart failure which was greater than that observed in the group of patients in whom digoxin was maintained (p=0.001). Digoxin withdrawal also significantly decreased exercise time and left ventricular ejection fraction. (From RADIANCE. N. Engl. J. Med. 1993;**329**:1.)

210 Effect of digoxin on survival. The Digitalis Investigator Group (DIG) study included patients with heart failure in sinus rhythm, functional class II–III and left ventricular ejection fraction <45%. The patients were treated with digoxin (n=3397) or placebo (n=3403), in addition to conventional therapy over a mean of 37 months (28–58 months). No differences in mortality were observed between the two treatment groups. (From DIG. *N. Engl. J. Med.* 1997;**336**:525.)

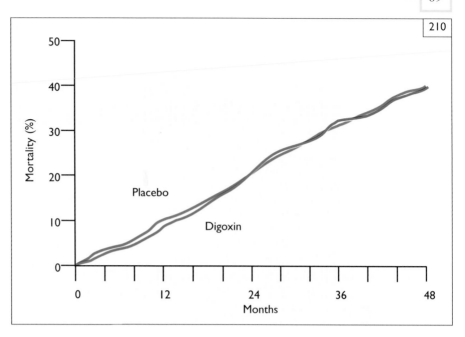

Table 33 Pharmacokinetic properties of digoxin			
Oral absorption (%)	60–75	Maximal effect (hours)	
Protein binding (%)	25	*i.v.*	2–4
Volume of distribution (l/kg)	6 (3–9)	*oral*	3–6
Half-life (hours)	36 (26–46)	Duration (days)	2–6
Elimination	Renal	Therapeutic level (ng/ml)	0.5–2.0
Onset (minutes)			
i.v.	5–30		
oral	30–90		

Oral absorption is 60–75% of the administered dose; when given by this route, maximal levels are reached after 30–90 minutes and its action is maximal after 3–6 h. When given i.v., onset of action is at 5–30 min and this reaches its maximum at 2–4 h.

It is approximately 25% bound to plasma proteins and is widely distributed through the body, crossing the blood brain barrier and the placenta. It accumulates in skeletal muscle, liver and heart, where it may reach concentrations that are 10 to 50 times higher than serum levels. This explains why haemodialysis eliminates little of the digoxin load in digoxin toxicity. Cardiac uptake of digoxin increases in patients with hypokalaemia and decreases in the presence of hyperkalaemia, hypercalcaemia or hypomagnesaemia. Digoxin undergoes very little biotransformation, and is mainly eliminated through glomerular filtration and somewhat by tubular secretion. In patients with renal insufficiency, the half-life of digoxin increases 2–4 times, so that the maintenance dose must be determined according to the creatinine clearance, generally requiring half of the usual dose and, in severe cases, intermittent dosing.

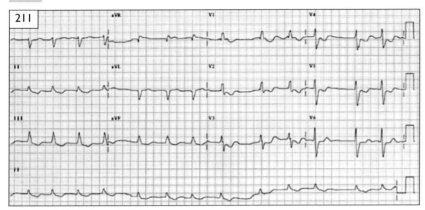

211 Electrocardiogram showing patient with chronic atrial fibrillation receiving long-term digoxin therapy. Widespread ST segment depression is evident.

Toxic effects of digoxin range from nausea and vomiting to xanthopsia (yellow discolouration of vision) and potentially lethal arrhythmias. Toxicity is exacerbated by concurrent hypokalaemia (a frequent finding in a diuretic-treated population), hypercalcaemia, or disthyroidism. Severe toxicity necessitates treatment with digoxin-specific antibody fragments (Digibind). Chronic treatment (but not necessarily toxicity) with digoxin may be associated with a typical 'reverse-tick' appearance of electrocardiographic ST segments (**211**).

SYMPATHOMIMETICS

These agents can be further classified according to their main pharmacological site of action: stimulation of α-, β_1-, β_2-adrenoceptors, or dopaminergic receptor subtype (*Table 34*).

Dopamine and dobutamine may act upon both adrenergic and dopaminergic receptors. Their pharmacological sites and clinical effects are shown in *Table 35*. Dobutamine (a synthetic agent) predominantly exerts a β_1 stimulatory effect, resulting in increased myocardial contractility. It has little effect upon dopaminergic receptors. In contrast, the endogenous catecholamine dopamine stimulates both adrenergic and dopaminergic receptors, depending upon dosage administered. For example, at lower doses dopaminergic receptor stimulation results in selective vasodilatation of the renal vascular bed, thought to result in increased renal perfusion. Higher doses invoke a β_1-mediated positive inotropic response, while further increases result in elevated systemic vascular resistance and heart rate. These agents are used in severe HF that is refractory to treatment with intravenous diuretics and vasodilators. Dobutamine has advantages over dopamine due to the relatively lower frequency of tachycardia and arrhythmias, although low-dose dopamine may contribute to improved renal blood flow and diuresis. However, meta-analysis of trials of intravenous inotropes has suggested a trend towards higher mortality.

The potential role of an oral dopamine analogue, ibopamine, was studied in the second Prospective Randomized Study of Ibopamine on Mortality and Efficacy (PRIME II) study. Ibopamine was associated with significantly higher mortality compared to placebo. Similarly, xamoterol, a partial agonist of the β_1 receptor, was associated with increased adverse events (all-cause mortality, deaths from progressive HF, and sudden deaths) compared to placebo in patients with moderate–severe HF.

Table 34 Classification of beta-adrenergic stimulants
β_1 Stimulants
Increase contractility
Butopamine, dobutamine, doxaminol, prenalterol, tazolol, xamoterol
β_2 Stimulants
Produce arterial vasodilatation and reduce SVR
Carbuterol, fenoterol, pirbuterol, quinterenol, rimiterol, salbutamol, salmefamol, soterenol, terbutaline, tretoquinol
Mixed
Dopamine
In an attempt to find options to digoxin, in the 1980s different positive inotropic drugs became available, among them beta-adrenergic agonists and phosphodiesterase III inhibitors. Both groups of drugs increase the intracellular concentration of cAMP; β-adrenergic agonists by stimulating the activity of adenylate cyclase, which converts ATP into cAMP, and the phosphodiesterase III inhibitors by inhibiting the breakdown of cAMP. The β-adrenergic agonists can be classified according to the capacity for stimulating the cardiac β_1 receptors (increasing contractility and heart rate), β_2-vasodilatory receptors, or both (mixed). SVR: systemic vascular resistance.

Phosphodiesterase inhibitors

Several inotropes exert their effect by increasing intracellular levels of cyclic adenosine monophosphate (cAMP). This 'second messenger' is degraded by the action of the enzyme phosphodiesterase. Milrinone and enoximone are examples which have been studied in chronic HF. These agents increase contractility and also promote vasodilatation ('inodilators'). Both drugs (administered orally) were associated with higher rates of mortality than placebo, with milrinone also causing more hospitalizations. Another oral inotrope, vesnarinone, acts as a phosphodiesterase inhibitor but also appears to enhance calcium influx. Following promising survival data from a study assessing vesnarinone in nearly 600 patients with HF, the VESnarinone Trial (VEST) recruited 3833 subjects with moderate–severe HF, with follow-up of 9.5 months. However, this trial was terminated early due to excess mortality in the treatment group.

Levosimendan is a relatively new inodilator that increases myofilament sensitivity to calcium, and has been shown to improve cardiac haemodynamics and symptoms in HF. The LIDO study compared levosimendan with dobutamine in patients hospitalized with severe (systolic) HF, thought to require invasive monitoring and intravenous inotropes. Levosimendan achieved significantly greater improvement in haemodynamic performance than dobutamine. In addition, although not the primary outcome, 6-month mortality was reduced with levosimendan. Future studies are needed to establish a role in treatment.

Summary

The last decade has provided a great deal of data confirming a role for β-blockade in HF. Increasingly widespread use may improve survival in HF, although previous practice advocating avoidance needs to be overcome. Inotropes, in contrast, do not appear to contribute to survival, and, indeed, may be harmful, although levosimendan has shown promising results in early trials. Digoxin therapy, at least, has not been associated with higher mortality, as opposed to other inotropes, and may reduce morbidity.

Table 35 Effects of dopamine and dobutamine

| | Dopamine (µg/kg/minute) | | | Dobutamine |
	<2	2–5	>5	
Receptors	DA_1/DA_2	β_1	$\beta_1 + \alpha$	β_1
Contractility	+/-	++	++	++
Heart rate	+/-	+	++	+/-
Arterial pressure	+/-	+	++	++
Renal perfusion	++	+	+/-	+
Arrhythmia	-	+/-	++	+/-

The haemodynamic effects vary, depending on the dose used:

Low doses (0.2–2 µg/kg/minute): dopamine stimulates DA_1 and DA_2 receptors, producing renal, mesenteric, cerebral, and coronary vasodilatation. Renal vasodilatation increases glomerular filtration rate, urine production, and renal excretion of Na; the majority of Na excretion seems to be due to a direct tubular action of dopamine and stimulation of DA_2 receptors that inhibit the liberation of aldosterone. Inhibition of sympathetic tone produced by the stimulation of DA_2 receptors explains why at these doses the arterial pressure decreases slightly and the heart rate remains the same or even falls. These doses are used for induction of diuresis, particularly in patients who do not respond to frusemide (furosemide).

Intermediate doses (2–5 µg/kg/minute): dopamine also stimulates cardiac β_1 and β_2 receptors, increasing contractility, heart rate and cardiac output at the same time as it decreases peripheral resistance (stimulation of DA_1 and β_2 receptors). These doses are used in the treatment of heart failure without hypotension.

High doses (>5 µg/kg/minute): dopamine also stimulates α-adrenergic receptors, increasing peripheral resistance and blood pressure. In addition, the marked stimulation of the cardiac β_1 receptors increases the heart rate and contractility, the myocardial O_2 demand, and may produce arrhythmias. These doses are only used in patients with severe hypotension and/or cardiogenic shock.

Further reading

The CIBIS II Investigators. The Cardiac Insufficiency Bisoprolol Study II (CIBIS-II): a randomized trial. *Lancet* 1999;**353**:9–13.

Cleland JG, Pennell DJ, Ray SG, *et al*. Carvedilol hibernating reversible ischaemia trial: marker of success investigators. Myocardial viability as a determinant of the ejection fraction response to carvedilol in patients with heart failure (CHRISTMAS trial): randomized controlled trial. *Lancet* 2003;**362**(9377):14–21.

Cleland JG, Nikitin N, McGowan J. Levosimendan: first in a new class of inodilator for acute and chronic severe heart failure. *Expert Rev. Cardiovasc. Ther.* 2004;**2**(1):9–19.

Hood WB Jr, Dans AL, Guyatt GH, Jaeschke R, McMurray JJ. Digitalis for treatment of congestive heart failure in patients in sinus rhythm: a systemic review and meta-analysis. *J. Cardiac Fail.* 2004;**10**(2):155–164.

The MERIT-HF Investigators. Effect of metoprolol CR/XL in chronic heart failure: Metoprolol CR/XL Randomized Intervention Trial in Congestive Heart Failure (MERIT-HF). *Lancet* 1999;**353**:2001–2007.

Packer M, Coats AJ, Fowler MB, *et al*. Effect of carvedilol on survival in severe chronic heart failure. *N. Engl. J. Med.*2001;**344**:1651–1658.

Poole-Wilson PA, Swedberg K, Cleland JG, *et al*. Carvedilol Or Metoprolol European Trial Investigators. Comparison of carvedilol and metoprolol on clinical outcomes in patients with chronic heart failure in the Carvedilol Or Metoprolol European Trial (COMET): randomized controlled trial. *Lancet* 2003;**362**(9377):7–13.

Chapter seven

Other vasodilators: nitrates and calcium channel blockers

Classification of vasodilators

Vasodilators may be classified according to the type of vessel predominantly affected (**212**). Further classification with respect to pharmacological mode of action may also be made. The major role of angiotensin-converting enzyme (ACE) inhibitors has been discussed in detail in Chapter 5. This chapter will focus upon the role of two other vasodilators, organic nitrates and calcium channel blockers, in heart failure (HF). These drugs already have well-established roles in the relief of angina and hypertension.

Principles of vasodilator therapy in heart failure

As discussed in Chapter 3, the syndrome of HF is associated with chronic neurohormonal activation, with the subsequent increase in systemic vascular resistance ultimately diminishing cardiac performance further. Direct arteriolar dilatation may be expected, therefore, to improve cardiac performance. As previously noted, the ability of the failing heart to adapt to increased preload (Frank–Starling relationship) is diminished. Venous dilatation reduces cardiac filling pressures by decreasing venous return.

212 Classification of vasodilators.

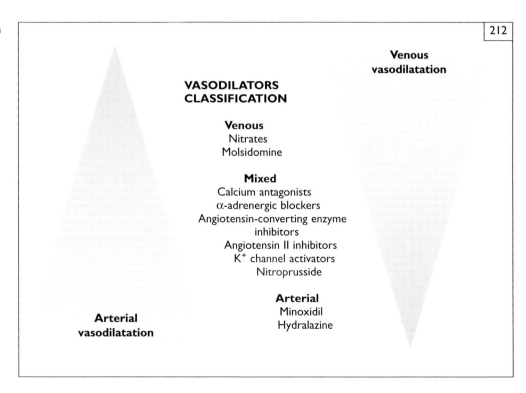

212

Venous vasodilatation

VASODILATORS CLASSIFICATION

Venous
Nitrates
Molsidomine

Mixed
Calcium antagonists
α-adrenergic blockers
Angiotensin-converting enzyme inhibitors
Angiotensin II inhibitors
K^+ channel activators
Nitroprusside

Arterial
Minoxidil
Hydralazine

Arterial vasodilatation

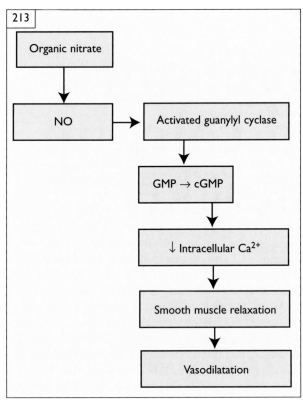

213 Mechanism of action of nitrates in smooth muscle cells. NO: nitric oxide; cGMP: cyclic guanosine monophosphate.

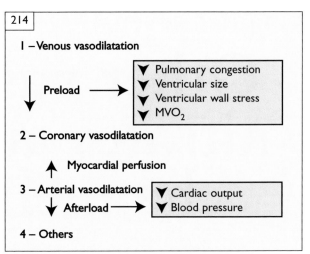

214 Haemodynamic effects of nitrates. At therapeutic doses, nitrates produce venodilatation that reduces systemic and pulmonary venous resistances. As a consequence, right atrial pressure, pulmonary capillary pressure, and left ventricular end-diastolic pressure (LVEDP) decrease. The preload reduction improves the signs of pulmonary congestion and decreases myocardial wall tension and ventricular size, which in turn reduce oxygen consumption (MVO_2). With higher doses, nitrates produce arterial vasodilatation that decreases peripheral vascular resistance and mean arterial pressure, leading to a decrease in afterload, and thereby reduce oxygen consumption. This arterial vasodilatation increases cardiac output, counteracting the possible reduction caused by the reduction in preload caused by venodilatation. The overall effect on cardiac output depends on the LVEDP; when LVEDP is high, nitrates increase cardiac output, while when it is normal nitrates can decrease cardiac output. Nitrates can also produce coronary vasodilatation, as much through reducing preload as through a direct effect on the vascular endothelium. This vasodilatation can decrease the mechanical compression of subendocardial vessels and increases blood flow at this level. Additionally, nitrates reduce coronary vascular tone, overcoming vasospasm.

Nitrates

Nitrates have been used in the symptomatic treatment of ischaemic heart disease for several decades. Modes of administration include short-acting, sublingual aerosol sprays, oral formulations with variable pharmacokinetics, transdermal preparations with longer duration of action, and intravenous agents. Nitrates have not been shown to improve survival in patients with chronic angina or with acute myocardial infarction (MI).

MECHANISM OF ACTION
Nitrates act principally as venodilators, and reduce left ventricular oxygen demand by reducing venous return, thereby relieving symptoms of angina. They are also highly effective coronary vasodilators. The reduction of ventricular preload is beneficial in those with dyspnoea resulting from left ventricular failure.

At the cellular level (**213**), upon entry into smooth muscle cells nitrates are metabolized to nitric oxide (NO). This molecule, in turn, activates the enzyme guanylyl cyclase, which catalyses the conversion of guanosine monophosphate (GMP) to cyclic GMP (cGMP). Cyclic GMP reduces intracellular calcium levels, which results in vasodilatation.

HAEMODYNAMIC BENEFITS
The effect of nitrate administration upon various haemodynamic parameters in the context of HF has been assessed in several studies (**214**). Venodilatation reduces ventricular preload, which has favourable consequences on pulmonary congestion, ventricular

dimensions, and wall stress. Arterial dilatation reduces ventricular afterload, resulting in increased cardiac output. Coronary vasodilatation may improve myocardial perfusion, which may be of particular benefit in hibernating myocardial regions, in which contractility may be increased. Additionally, nitrates may have beneficial effects on mitral valve regurgitation. Left ventricular remodelling results in dilatation of the ventricle, with associated dilatation of the mitral valve annulus. Progressive annular dilatation results in valve regurgitation, which has the capacity to worsen cardiac function further. Nitrates have been shown to reduce mitral valve regurgitant area.

NITRATES AND HEART FAILURE

Despite the benefits described above, the impact of nitrate therapy alone upon survival in HF has not been evaluated. Instead, two moderately large, prospective, randomized-controlled studies have studied the role of oral nitrates (specifically isosorbide dinitrate, ISDN) when combined with hydralazine, predominantly an arteriolar vasodilator. These studies, the Vasodilators in Heart Failure Trials (V-HeFT), were conducted in American men before and after the demonstration of significant benefits resulting from the use of ACE inhibitors in HF.

The first study recruited 642 subjects with mild–moderate HF, who were already receiving diuretic and digoxin therapy; 273 patients received placebo, while 186 received the hydralazine–nitrate combination (target doses of 75mg qds and 40mg qds for hydralazine and ISDN, respectively). The remaining 183 received the α-adrenoceptor antagonist prazosin. Survival with prazosin was no different to placebo. However, treatment with the hydralazine–nitrate combination was associated with significantly improved survival after 2 years of follow-up (**215**). The overall improved survival was of borderline significance, but this study provided the basis for VHeFT II, which compared the same vasodilator combination with the ACE inhibitor enalapril. Of note, 19% of patients discontinued one or both of hydralazine or ISDN due to side-effects, mainly headache and dizziness.

VHeFT II recruited 800 men with predominantly mild-moderate HF; half received the vasodilator combination used in VHeFT I, whereas the remainder received enalapril (aiming for a dose of 20 mg OD). The hydralazine–ISDN combination was associated with significantly greater improvements in left ventricular ejection fraction (LVEF) and exercise tolerance than enalapril. However, 2-year mortality was significantly lower in the group treated with the

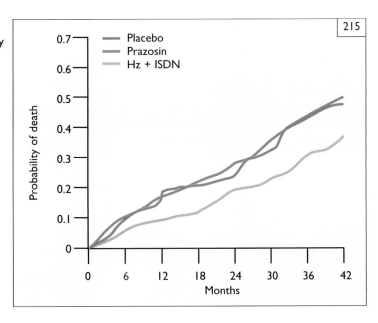

215 Nitrates and survival (VHeFT-I). In men with class II–III heart failure, the VHeFT-I study showed that for patients already treated with digoxin and diuretics, the combination of hydralazine (Hz; 300 mg/day) and isosorbide dinitrate (ISDN; 160 mg/day) (n=186) improved symptoms and functional status. More importantly, combination therapy was associated with a 23% reduction in mortality at 3 years; this effect was not seen in patients treated with prazosin (30 mg/day) (n=183). Selection of the treatment arms in this study was based on certain suppositions. The placebo group (n=273) received digitalis and diuretics, and subsequent to this study the combination has been administered obligatorily in control groups. The combined administration of hydralazine (arterial vasodilator) and a nitrate (venodilator) was designed to provide equilibrated vasodilatation. Prazosin combined both arterial and venous vasodilatory capacities in one medication, and was initially assumed to be better than combination therapy. The lack of effect of prazosin was probably due to development of tolerance. Perhaps the most relevant finding of the study was that, in practice, the effects of a medicine on symptoms or haemodynamic effects do not correlate well with effects on overall survival. (From VHefT-I. *N. Engl. J. Med.* 1986;**314**:1547.)

ACE inhibitor, due to lower incidence of sudden death (**216**). Again, adherence to combination therapy was low: 29% and 31 % had discontinued hydralazine and ISDN, respectively, whereas 22% had discontinued enalapril.

Subsequent retrospective analysis of the VHeFT II data has revealed possible benefit of hydralazine–ISDN among black patients, who may not respond to ACE inhibition as well as white counterparts. This potential has been prospectively evaluated in the African-American Heart Failure Trial (AHeFT), which compared the hydralazine–ISDN combination with placebo in African-Americans with NYHA III–IV HF with LVEF <35% on standard therapy including ACE inhibitors. This trial was stopped early due to a significant mortality benefit in the hydralazine–ISDN group. The place of this drug in other populations remains unclear.

At present, ACE inhibitors remain the vasodilator of choice; hydralazine and nitrates may be considered in those intolerant to ACE inhibitors, although this indication has not been definitively evaluated. Furthermore, the combination is associated with relatively poor compliance, owing to frequent side-effects.

NITRATE RESISTANCE AND TOLERANCE
To compound the evident limited tolerability of nitrates when used in combination with hydralazine, experience shows that their usefulness is further reduced by resistance and by development of tolerance. Patients receiving longer acting nitrate preparations (especially transdermally) develop tolerance rapidly (**217**), but tolerance can develop with all nitrates, and is dose-dependent.

Previous studies have shown that resistance may be related to the presence of higher right atrial pressures associated with fluid overload. Vessels that are already distended, therefore, may be prevented from dilating further in response to nitrates. Alternatively, decompensation could lead to intestinal mucosal oedema and impairment of oral nitrate absorption. Similarities between nitrate resistance and endothelial dysfunction, common in patients with HF, are also apparent; raised circulating levels of catecholamines, angiotensin II, and endothelin have been implicated. The mechanisms underlying nitrate tolerance are not clear. Evidence points to production of the superoxide radical (O_2^-), which may be liberated by a dysfunctional endothelium, or may be mediated by nitrates themselves. A separate mechanism may relate to impairment of metabolic pathways that produce NO from organic nitrates (abnormal nitrate biotransformation).

Practical measures to reduce nitrate tolerance include employing dosage regimes that permit a drop in plasma nitrate levels (e.g. for 4–8 hours) and using the lowest effective dose. The ability of adjunctive agents such as ACE inhibitors, N-acetylcysteine, and folic acid to improve nitrate efficacy has been studied, but these agents have not been shown to reduce nitrate tolerance definitively.

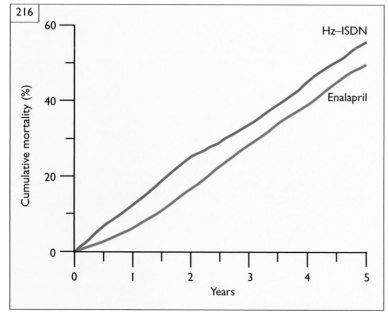

216 Nitrates and survival (VHeFT-II). The angiotensin-converting enzyme inhibitor enalapril is associated with decreased mortality when compared with hydralazine–isosorbide dinitrate (Hz–ISDN) in patients with moderate NYHA II–III heart failure (18% versus 25%, p=0.016 at 2 years; 48% versus 54%, p=0.08 at 5 years). (From Cohn JN, et al. N. Engl. J. Med. 1991;**325**:303.)

217 Nitrates and tolerance. Tolerance is related to the duration of the nitrate effects, such that the longer the half-life, the higher the risk that tolerance will occur. ISDN: isosorbide dinitrate; ISMN: isosorbide mononitrate; GTN: glyceryl trinitrate; s.l.: sublingual.

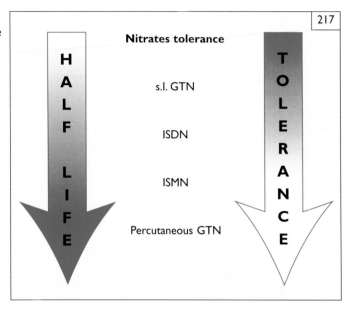

NICORANDIL

Nicorandil is a potent coronary and peripheral vasodilator with a dual mechanism of action. In addition to a nitrate-like action, nicorandil also functions as a potassium channel opener. It is increasingly used to relieve angina, and the Impact Of Nicorandil in Angina (IONA) study reported improved outcome in patients with stable angina treated with nicorandil, compared to placebo.

Although no long-term studies have evaluated its efficacy and safety in HF, some small studies have noted benefits. For example, intravenous administration in patients with moderate–severe HF produced longer-lasting haemodynamic improvements than those obtained with intravenous nitroglycerin. Animal studies have reported an attenuation of ventricular dilatation when oral nicorandil is administered following reperfused MI. Future studies may provide evidence of further benefits.

Calcium channel blockers

Calcium channel blockers (CCBs) are used in the treatment of a variety of cardiovascular disorders including hypertension, ischaemic heart disease, supraventricular tachycardia, and subarachnoid haemorrhage. Their effects include arterial vasodilatation, reduction in myocardial contractility, reduction in heart rate, and impairment in conduction, with overall effects depending on the properties of individual agents.

Table 36 Classification of calcium channel blockers

Phenylalkylamines
◇ Verapamil: marked negative inotrope

Benzothiazepines
◇ Diltiazem: moderate negative inotrope

Dihydropyridines: predominant vasodilatory effects
◇ Nifedipine: mild negative inotrope in heart failure
◇ Nimodipine
◇ Nicardipine
◇ Amlodipine
◇ Felodipine

CLASSIFICATION AND MECHANISM OF ACTION

CCBs can be divided according to chemical group (*Table 36*). Their mechanism of action relates to their blocking of calcium channels within smooth muscle cells and cardiac tissue. They principally block the L-type calcium channel, also known as the slow conduction channel. These channels permit the influx of calcium, which facilitates myocardial contraction and vasoconstriction, and is responsible for the plateau phase of the action potential within conducting tissues. CCBs reduce intracellular calcium levels, leading to vasodilatation and slowing electrical recovery of conducting tissue.

Verapamil has a negative inotropic action, making it less suitable for use in patients with left ventricular systolic dysfunction. This also applies to diltiazem, although the reduction in contractility is relatively less marked. In particular, verapamil should not be used in conjunction with β-blockers. Both of these agents have a negative chronotropic effect, and can reduce conduction within the sino-atrial and atrio-ventricular nodes.

Essentially, the dihydropyridines possess the greatest vasodilating properties with, at most, mild negatively inotropic properties. They also have relatively little effect on heart rate and conduction. Arterial vasodilatation reduces peripheral resistance, making them useful in the treatment of hypertension. Additionally, coronary vasodilatation (and negative chronotropy) enable CCBs to relieve angina. The reduction in peripheral vascular resistance also reduces left ventricular impedance and, therefore, CCBs which are not negatively inotropic have been evaluated in the treatment of HF.

CALCIUM CHANNEL BLOCKERS AND HEART FAILURE
Although verapamil, diltiazem and, to a lesser extent, nifedipine depress myocardial contractility, this does not apply to amlodipine. This dihydropyridine has been evaluated in large HF trials that addressed morbidity and mortality. Small studies of short duration noted symptomatic and functional improvement in subjects treated with amlodipine, and this led to larger studies.

The first Prospective Randomized Amlodipine Survival Evaluation (PRAISE) study recruited over 1100 patients with moderate–severe HF (and LVEF <30%), and administered either placebo or amlodipine in addition to diuretics, ACE inhibitors and digoxin. The trial included 421 patients with nonischaemic cardiomyopathy, and median follow-up extended to 14 months. Combined risk of fatal and nonfatal events was reduced by amlodipine in the nonischaemic group, whereas it was no different to placebo in those with ischaemic cardiomyopathy. Overall, amlodipine was well tolerated; pulmonary oedema was more frequent in the amlodipine group, but the overall worsening of HF did not differ between the two groups. Uncontrolled hypertension was less common in the treatment group. Amlodipine, like other CCBs, has the tendency to cause peripheral oedema, which may confuse the clinical picture in HF.

The apparent survival advantage in the small number of patients with nonischaemic cardiomyopathy was assessed further in the subsequent PRAISE II study. However, initial results showed no difference in outcome between the treatment and placebo groups.

Neither felodipine nor diltiazem has been associated with improved survival in the small randomized-controlled trials assessing their respective efficacies. Furthermore, felodipine did not improve morbidity or mortality in the 450 men with chronic HF recruited into VHeFT-III.

Summary
Currently, therefore, nitrates do not have a role in standard HF therapy. In combination with hydralazine, they may be useful in patients unable to tolerate ACE inhibitors or angiotensin receptor blockers. Whether nitrates possess additive benefits to blockade of the renin–angiotensin–aldosterone system is not clear at present. CCBs should not be used to treat HF, and the negatively inotropic agents should be avoided altogether. Amlodipine has a neutral effect upon mortality in HF, and may be of value in the treatment of associated hypertension in addition to ACE inhibition and β-blockade.

Further reading
Cohn JN, Archibald DG, Ziesche S, et al. Effect of vasodilator therapy on mortality in chronic congestive heart failure. Results of a Veterans Administration Cooperative Study. N. Engl. J. Med. 1986;314:1547–1552.

Cohn JN, Johnson G, Ziesche S, et al. A comparison of enalapril with hydralazine-isosorbide dinitrate in the treatment of chronic congestive heart failure. N. Engl. J. Med. 1991;325:303–310.

Gori T, Parker JD. The puzzle of nitrate tolerance: pieces smaller than we thought? Circulation 2002;106:2404–2408.

Gori T, Parker JD. Nitrate tolerance: a unifying hypothesis. Circulation 2002;106:2510–2513.

The Prospective Randomized Amlodipine Survival Evaluation (PRAISE) Study Group. Effect of amlodipine on morbidity and mortality in severe chronic heart failure. N. Engl. J. Med. 1996;335:1107–1114.

Chapter eight

Antiarrhythmic and antithrombotic therapy in heart failure

Introduction

The preceding chapters have focused on therapies directed at the syndrome of heart failure (HF) itself, designed to ameliorate symptoms or enhance myocardial function. However, much of the morbidity and mortality related to HF occurs as a result of thrombotic (coronary thrombosis, stroke, venous thromboembolism) or arrhythmic (sudden cardiac death, atrial fibrillation) complications. This chapter will review the place of antiarrhythmic and antithrombotic medication in HF (*Table 37*). Device therapy for arrhythmia is covered in Chapter 9.

Antiarrhythmic drug therapy in heart failure

ATRIAL FIBRILLATION

Atrial fibrillation (AF) is common in patients with HF, affecting 10–50%. The onset of AF in a patient previously in sinus rhythm (SR) is a common cause of admission to hospital, either due to symptomatic palpitations, or due to decompensation of previously controlled HF.

Class	Mechanism	Example
I	Sodium channel blockers	
Ia	Action potential prolonged	Quinidine
Ib	Action potential shortened	Lignocaine
Ic	Action potential unchanged	Flecainide
II	β-blockers	Bisoprolol, carvedilol
III	Blockade of potassium channels, prolong repolarization	Amiodarone, dofetilide, sotalol (Class II, III actions)
IV	Nondihydropyridine calcium antagonists	Verapamil, diltiazem

Table 37 Vaughan-Williams classification of antiarrhythmic drugs

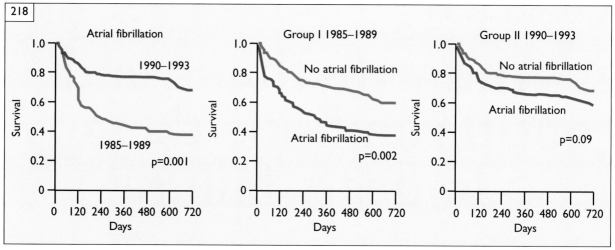

218 Effect of atrial fibrillation on mortality in CHF may be decreasing, demonstrated by this comparative study. Benefits may well be due to increasing use of anticoagulation in these patients. (From Stevenson WG, et al. J. Am. Coll. Cardiol. 1996;**28**:1458.)

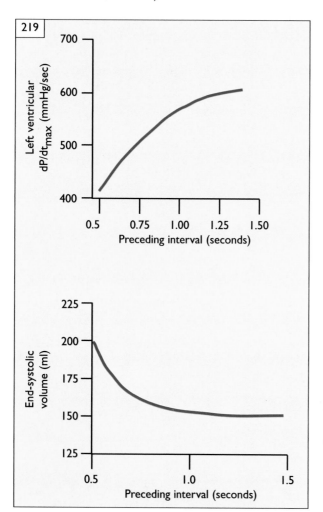

219 Contractility is improved by rate control in rapid atrial fibrillation. (From Brookes CI, et al. Circulation 1998;**98**:1762.)

Mortality is higher in HF patients with AF than those in sinus rhythm (**218**), although recent studies suggest this effect is decreasing. AF is associated with adverse haemodynamic effects, including reduction of the left ventricular ejection fraction (LVEF) by as much as 10%. This may represent a highly significant reduction in systolic function, particularly in patients with preexisting impairment of left ventricular (LV) function. Although resolution of AF is associated with improvement in LV function, simply controlling the ventricular rate also improves LV function (**219**); several recent studies (including patients with impairment of LV function) suggest that aggressive rhythm control does not reduce mortality when compared with a rate control and anticoagulation strategy in AF. Additionally, patients with structural heart disease such as dilated left atrium or mitral valve disease are less likely to revert to SR with electrical or pharmacological cardioversion. Therefore, in most patients with HF complicated by AF, the goal should be to control the ventricular rate.

Digoxin is frequently used for control of ventricular rate in patients with AF. However, it is poor at controlling ventricular rate during exertion, limiting its usefulness in patients with HF where one goal is increased functional capacity. It must also be used with caution in patients with renal impairment, a common finding in severe HF.

β-blockers may be used in the treatment of AF. β-blockers may help to maintain SR in patients with paroxysmal AF, and are more effective than digoxin at controlling ventricular rate in persistent AF. However, the doses needed to control adequately the

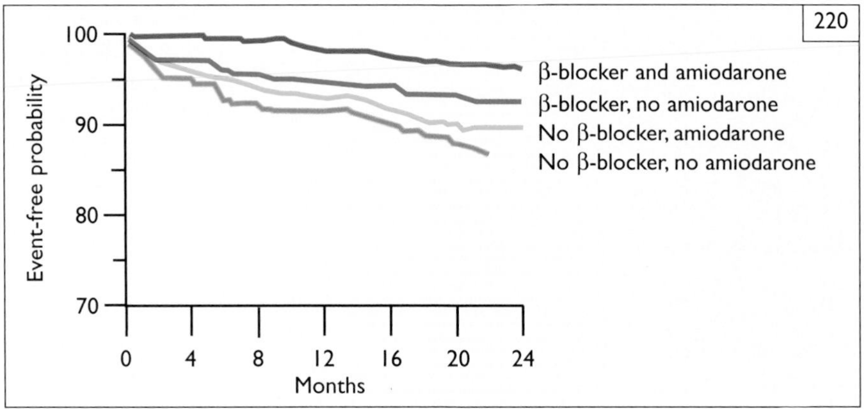

220 Data from the EMIAT and CAMIAT trials suggested that amiodarone and β blockade together may have additive beneficial effect on mortality in post-MI patients. CAMIAT: Canadian Amiodarone Myocardial Infarction Arrhythmia Trial; EMIAT: European Amiodarone Myocardial Infarction Arrhythmia Trial; MI: myocardial infarction. (From Boutitie F, *et al. Circulation* 1999;**99**:2268.)

Table 38 Side-effects of amiodarone

- ✧ Photosensitivity
- ✧ Slate-grey skin pigmentation (see **70**)
- ✧ Pulmonary fibrosis
- ✧ Corneal microdeposits
- ✧ Peripheral neuropathy
- ✧ Hypo- or hyperthyroidism
- ✧ Abnormalities of liver function

ventricular rate may be higher than some patients are able to tolerate.The need to introduce β-blockers slowly in this patient population limits their usefulness in the acute situation.

Amiodarone may be used to control AF acutely. Intravenous (via a central venous line) or oral loading may be used depending upon the clinical situation. The usual maintainence dose of 200 mg daily is often sufficient to control AF in the long term, although some patients may be able to discontinue amiodarone once β-blockers have been titrated up to an antiarrhythmic dose (220). This approach avoids the serious long-term side-effects of amiodarone (*Table 38*). Amiodarone may affect levels of other common drugs used in HF, notably warfarin and digoxin. Close monitoring of the international normalized ratio (INR), together with an approximate halving of the dose of warfarin, is needed when commencing amiodarone. Dofetilide, a new class III antiarrhythmic agent, may be an alternative to amiodarone for the control of AF (221). Both amiodarone and dofetilide may prolong the QTc interval, with an associated risk of torsade de pointes ventricular tachycardia.

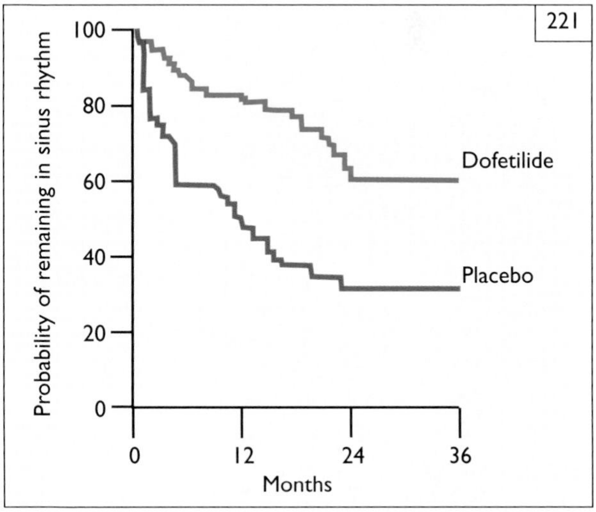

221 Results of the DIAMOND-CHF study – a subgroup of patients who were in atrial fibrillation at randomization and reverted to sinus rhythm; dofetilide increased the probability of maintaining sinus rhythm. (Dofetilide-treated patients who were in atrial fibrillation at randomization were also more likely to revert to sinus rhythm than those on placebo – data not shown.) (From Torp-Pedersen C, *et al. N. Engl. J. Med.* 1999;**341**:857.)

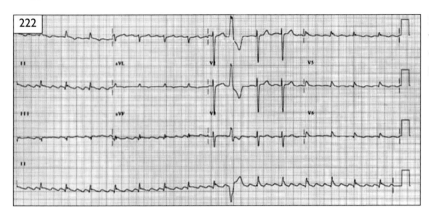

222 ECG showing atrial flutter with 2:1 block. Note the characteristic saw-tooth baseline pattern best seen in lead II.

Atrial flutter (**222**) is less common than AF, but may occur in HF, and has similar adverse effects to AF. Atrial flutter is less responsive to antiarrhythmic drugs, and a trial of direct current cardioversion may be more worthwhile than in AF. Control of AF or flutter may sometimes require combinations of the above drugs. In some patients, AF may remain uncontrolled despite the use of multiple drugs; in such cases, ablation of the atrio-ventricular node with pacemaker insertion may improve symptoms and cardiac function (**223**).

MALIGNANT VENTRICULAR ARRHYTHMIAS AND SUDDEN
CARDIAC DEATH
Prevention
The recognition that many patients with HF die suddenly led to the idea that prophylactic anti-arrhythmic medication might improve survival. Multiple trials using a variety of therapeutic agents have been performed. β-blockers have been shown to reduce mortality and sudden cardiac death (SCD), and are recommended for all patients with symptomatic HF, as reviewed in Chapter 6. Results of trials of other antiarrhythmic agents has been less convincing.

Trials of class I antiarrhythmic drugs such as flecainide in ischaemic heart disease (such as the Cardiac Arrhythmia Suppression Trial [CAST], which randomized postmyocardial infarction patients, including patients with HF, to flecainide or encainide versus placebo) showed increased mortality in the treatment group, and so these drugs are not recommended in HF (**224**). Post MI, amiodarone appears to reduce sudden death (**225**) Trials involving amiodarone have been conflicting. The Grupo de Estudio de la Sobrevida en Insuficiencia Cardíaca en Argentina (GESICA) trial involving over 500 patients with class III–IV HF found decreased mortality with amiodarone added to digoxin, diuretics, and angiotensin-converting

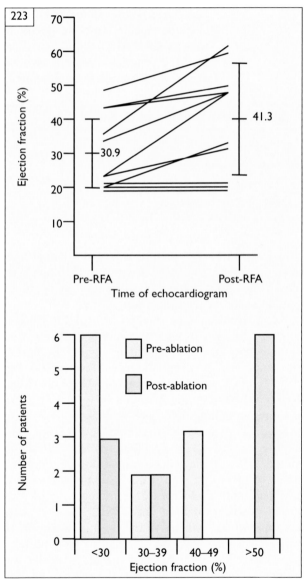

223 Restoration of sinus rhythm by radiofrequency ablation (RFA) in patients with chronic atrial flutter and cardiomyopathy improves left ventricular function. (From Luchsinger JA. *J. Am. Coll. Cardiol.* 1998;**32**:205–210.)

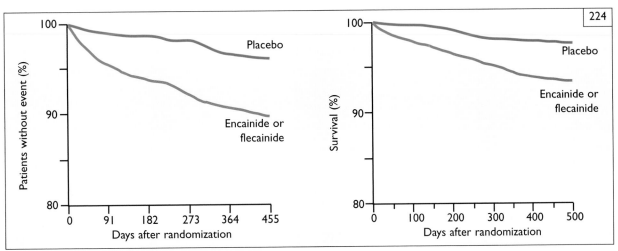

224 Results of the CAST trial. Class 1 antiarrythmic agents flecainide and encainide were associated with increased mortality in post-MI patients (including patients with CHF). CAST: Cardiac Arryhtmia Suppression Trial; MI: myocardial infarction. (From Echt DS, *et al. N. Engl. J. Med.* 1991;**324**:781.)

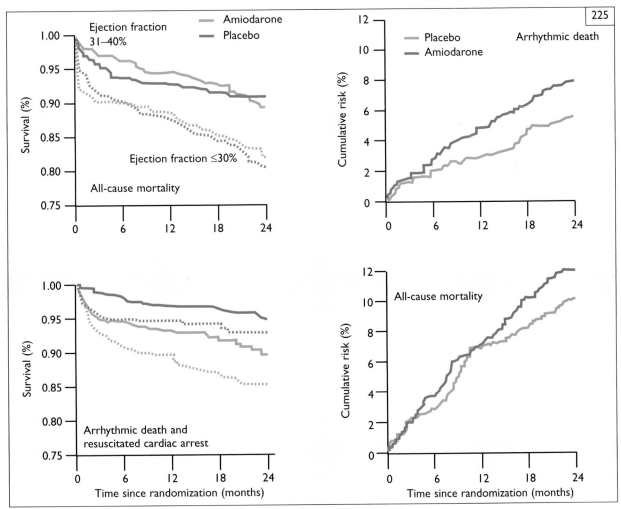

225 Summary of the EMIAT and CAMIAT trials of amiodarone post-myocardial infarction – no effect on all cause mortality. EMIAT: European Amiodarone Myocardial Infarction Arrhythmia Trial; CAMIAT: Canadian Amiodarone Myocardial Infarction Arrhythmia Trial. (From Julian DG, *et al. Lancet* 1997;**349**:667; Cairns JA, *et al. Lancet* 1997;**349**:675.)

enzyme (ACE) inhibitors. However, the Congestive Heart Failure Survival Trial of Antiarrhythmic Therapy (CHF-STAT) showed no improvement in mortality with amiodarone (*Table 39*). Meta-analyses of trials of amiodarone have suggested reductions in sudden death with amiodarone in HF. However, the recent SCD-HeFT trial (see Chapter 9) of implantable cardioverter defibrillators (ICD) in HF also randomized patients to amiodarone or placebo. No mortality benefit of amiodarone was seen, whereas a significant mortality reduction with ICD was found.

Treatment

It is not uncommon for a patient with HF to present to the emergency department with palpitations or decompensation, and for ventricular tachycardia to be found on electrocardiogram (ECG) monitoring. Equally, patients admitted with HF may experience malignant ventricular arrhythmias during their hospital admission. Such episodes should be treated according to resuscitation guidelines with DC cardioversion and adjunctive drugs, although the prognosis for patients with severe HF in this situation is very poor. All patients surviving such an episode should have serial ECGs and cardiac enzymes/troponin estimation to exclude myocardial infarction (MI).

Table 39 Comparison of GESICA and CHF-STAT studies

Trial	Reference	Patients	Aetiology	Treatment	Mean follow-up	Outcome
GESICA (Argentina)	*Lancet* 1994;**344**:493	516 (80% NYHA III–IV)	40% IHD 30% Alcohol 20% DCM 10% Chagas disease	Open label Amiodarone 600 mg/day for 14 days; 300 mg/day or no additional treatment	13 months	Mortality -28% risk reduction Admission -31% risk reduction
CHF-STAT (USA)	*N. Engl. J. Med.* 1995;**333**:77	674 (40% NYHA III–IV)	72% IHD 28% DCM	Blinded Amiodarone 800 mg/day for 14 days; 600 mg/day for 50 weeks; 300 mg/day or placebo	45 months	No improvement in survival No reduction in sudden death Increased LVEF

CHF-STAT: Congestive Heart Failure Survival Trial of Antiarrhythmic Therapy; DCM: dilated cardiomyopathy; GESICA: Grupo de Estudio de la Sobrevida en Insuficiencia Cardiaca en Argentina; IHD: ischaemic heart disease; LVEF: left ventricular ejection fraction; NYHA: New York Heart Association.

Recurrence of arrhythmia is common, and attention to contributing factors to reduce the risk is important. Low potassium or magnesium levels may contribute to the development of such arrhythmias, and should be corrected aggressively. Antiarrhythmic drugs (such as digoxin) may themselves be the cause of the arrhythmia, and careful review of the patient's medication list (and blood drug levels where appropriate) is essential. Patients suffering such an arrhythmia outside of the acute context of an MI may be candidates for an ICD (Chapter 9).

Antithrombotic therapy

As discussed in Chapter 2, patients with HF are at high risk of venous thromboembolism and stroke (*Table 40*), irrespective of the underlying aetiology. In addition, SCD, which occurs commonly in patients with HF, may be at least partly explained by thrombotic episodes such as pulmonary embolism or MI (**226**). Postmortem studies have consistently shown that victims of SCD commonly (>50%) demonstrate fresh coronary thrombus and/or occlusion (**227–229**). HF fulfils all the requirements of

Table 40 Stroke risk in major heart failure trials

Trial	Reference	Inclusion criteria	Stroke risk (%)
CONSENSUS	*N. Engl. J. Med.* 1987;**316**:1429	NYHA IV	4.6
PROMISE	*J. Am. Coll. Cardiol.* 1993;**21**:218A	NYHA III/IV, EF <35%	3.5
SAVE	*N. Engl. J. Med.* 1997;**336**:310	EF <40% post-MI	1.5
SOLVD	*Am. J. Cardiol.* 1997;**79**:909	EF <35% AF excluded	1.3
VHeFT-I, VHeFT-II	*Circulation* 1993;**87**(suppl VI):VI94	Impaired LV function	2.0, 1.9

AF: atrial fibrillation; EF: ejection fraction; LV: left ventricle; MI: myocardial infarction; NYHA: New York Heart Association. (For Trials see Appendix A.)

226 Pulmonary angiogram showing oligaemic lung fields and a filling defect within the pulmonary artery (arrow), due to pulmonary embolism.

227 Left ventricular angiogram showing a filling defect due to intraventricular thrombus (arrows).

228, 229 Echocardiogram showing apical thrombus (arrow).

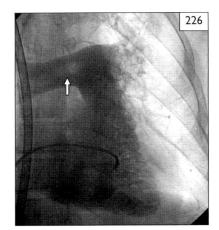

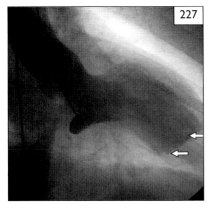

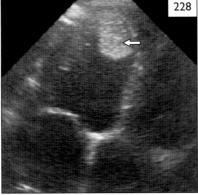

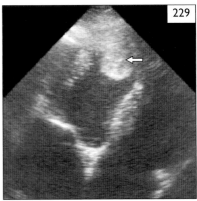

Virchow's triad for a prothrombotic state: abnormal flow (low cardiac output, dilated cardiac chambers), abnormal blood constituents (abnormal platelet structure and function), and abnormal vessel wall (endothelial dysfunction). In addition, as discussed above, antiarrhythmic drugs have consistently failed to show mortality benefit in HF, and even ICDs (Chapter 9) do not eliminate SCD in HF, suggesting that not all such deaths are arrhythmic.

PATIENTS WITH ATRIAL FIBRILLATION

As noted previously, AF is a common finding among patients with HF or asymptomatic LV dysfunction. AF is an important risk factor for stroke (**230**). Patients with AF and LV dysfunction are at higher risk of stroke than patients with AF alone, and the prognosis for patients with stroke is worse in the presence of LV dysfunction. It is widely accepted that all patients with AF and evidence of LV impairment without contraindications should receive dose-adjusted warfarin. Aspirin may provide some protection, and should be considered where warfarin is refused or contraindicated.

PATIENTS WITH INTRAVENTRICULAR THROMBUS

Patients with HF, particularly in the presence of recent MI or LV aneurysm, may develop intra-ventricular thrombus (see **227**). Clinical studies in patients with both ischaemic and nonischaemic cardiomyopathy suggest that the rate of thrombo-embolism in patients with echocardiographic evidence of mural thrombus is 5.3–7.0 per 100 patient years, which represents a two- to threefold increase over studies of HF populations as a whole. Anticoagulation with warfarin in such patients is recommended, particularly if there is any history of transient ischaemic episodes.

USE OF LONG-TERM ANTITHROMBOTIC AGENTS

Warfarin

Thus far, there is no clear evidence that warfarin is beneficial in patients with chronic HF in sinus rhythm, although it is accepted that all patients with AF and impaired LV function benefit from oral anticoagulation (*Table 41*). Most of the data concerning warfarin use in chronic HF come from retrospective, nonrandomized studies of large HF trials, which must be interpreted with caution. The Studies of Left Ventricular Dysfunction (SOLVD) showed no reduction in thromboembolic risk associated with warfarin use, but did find a significant reduction in sudden and overall cardiovascular death in those taking warfarin (**231**).

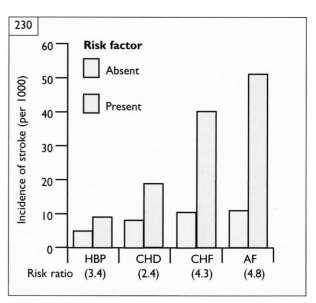

230 2-year age-adjusted risk of stroke in patients with hypertension (HBP), coronary heart disease (CHD), chronic heart failure (CHF) and atrial fibrillation (AF). (From Wolf PA, *et al. Stroke* 1991; **22**: 983–988.)

Table 41 Role of warfarin for chronic heart failure in sinus rhythm
LV aneurysm 3 months or more after acute MI
◇ Usually no need for echocardiogram or anticoagulation treatment, unless established chronic HF, intracardiac thrombus, or severe cardiac impairment present
Acute myocardial infarction
◇ Large MI, with associated congestive cardiac failure
◇ Anterior MI without heart failure, if LV thrombi are found on 2D echocardiography
Dilated cardiomyopathy
◇ Treatment with anticoagulants may be beneficial regardless of presence or absence of LV thrombi
Hypertrophic cardiomyopathy
◇ Treatment with anticoagulants not established, unless mural thrombus present or previous thromboembolic episode
HF: heart failure; LV: left ventricular; MI: myocardial infarction. (From Lip G. *Postgrad. Med. J.* 1996; **72**: 731–738.)

The Cooperative North Scandinavian Enalapril Survival study (CONSENSUS) found that patients taking warfarin had a 40% lower mortality than those not on anticoagulant therapy. Stroke was 81% lower in those taking warfarin in the Survival and Ventricular Enlargement (SAVE) study.

In contrast to these studies, the first Vasodilators in Heart Failure (VHeFT-I) study found no difference with anticoagulation and, surprisingly, VHeFT-II found a significantly increased risk of thromboembolism in the anticoagulated patients. In addition to these retrospective analyses, there have been a number of small observational studies of anticoagulants in HF, which have shown similarly conflicting results.

Antiplatelet agents
Although aspirin is used routinely in the post-MI setting, and in low-risk patients with AF, to date there is no published evidence from prospective, randomized trials on the use of antiplatelet agents in chronic HF. Such trials are underway (see below), but currently only observational data are available from further retrospective analyses of major HF trials. The SAVE study showed a 56% reduction in stroke risk with aspirin, with greater benefit in patients with worse LV function, and also showed a reduction in SCD for patients on aspirin. Aspirin also appeared to benefit the patients in the VHeFT studies, in contrast to anticoagulant therapy.

Prospective trials
The WATCH (Warfarin and Antiplatelet Therapy in Chronic Heart failure) study had a three arm design, comparing warfarin, clopidogrel (an inhibitor of platelet aggregation induced by adenosine diphosphate), and aspirin in patients with NYHA class II–IV symptoms and LVEF <35%. The study was stopped due to poor recruitment and there was no difference in primary endpoint of this study (composite of death, stroke, and MI). Meanwhile, the ongoing WARCEF (Warfarin Aspirin Reduced Cardiac Ejection Fraction) study is recruiting patients with NYHA I–III symptoms and LVEF <30%, and randomizing to either aspirin or warfarin with a primary combined endpoint of death and nonfatal stroke. The outcome of this trial is awaited with interest.

In addition, the new orally active, direct thrombin inhibitor ximelagatran may, in the future, be an alternative to warfarin in chronic HF. Ximelagatran may be more acceptable to patients, as it does not require coagulation monitoring or dose adjustment. Ximelagatran has been shown to be similarly effective as warfarin at preventing stroke in AF in the SPORTIF III study. However, ximelagatran may cause abnormal liver function requiring withdrawal.

COMPLICATIONS
Patients receiving antithrombotic therapy have an increased risk of bleeding, particularly those taking warfarin. This is frequently compounded in HF by the use of drugs which potentiate warfarin (such as amiodarone), and by hepatic dysfunction in decompensated HF. Careful monitoring of the INR is vital at initiation of therapy, and if any interacting

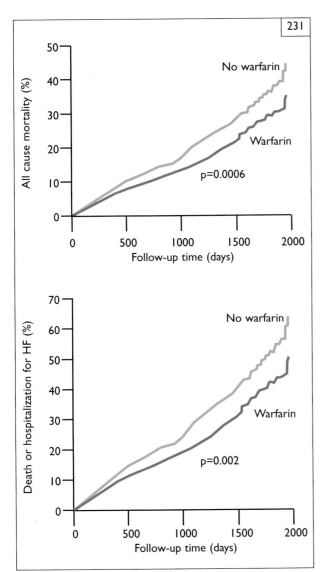

231 Results from the Studies of Left Ventricular Dysfunction (SOLVD) – reduced mortality in patients taking warfarin. (From Al-Khadna AS, *et al. J. Am. Coll. Cardiol.* 1998; **31**: 749–753.)

drug is started while the patient is taking warfarin (such as erythromycin for an intercurrent respiratory tract infection). Commonly interacting drugs are listed in *Table 42*.

Patients with bleeding diathesis, or who are at high risk of serious bleeding due to gastrointestinal ulceration or frequent falls, are unlikely to benefit from anticoagulation.

RECOMMENDATIONS

A high rate of thromboembolic complications contributes to the high morbidity and poor prognosis in HF. Many deaths in chronic HF are due to SCD which may have a thrombotic basis. Chronic HF satisfies all the requirements of Virchow's triad for a prothrombotic state, and therefore it would seem intuitive that antithrombotic therapy would provide these patients with significant morbidity and mortality benefit.

However, the evidence to date has been conflicting. The outcome of ongoing prospective studies may provide definitive guidance, but until this evidence is available, the decision to use long-term antithrombotic therapy must be made on a case-by-case basis.

Patients with HF rendered immobile by intercurrent illness are at very high risk of thromboembolism, and so short-term treatment with subcutaneous heparin according to local protocols is advised in this situation.

Further reading

Amiodarone trials meta-analysis investigators. Effect of prophylactic amiodarone on mortality after acute myocardial infarction and in congestive heart failure: meta-analysis of individual data from 6500 patients in randomized trials. *Lancet* 1997;**350**:1417–1424.

Echt DS, Liebson PR, Mitchell LB, *et al*. Mortality and morbidity in patients receiving encainide, flecainide, or placebo. The Cardiac Arrhythmia Suppression Trial. *N. Engl. J. Med.* 1991;**324**:781–788.

Elming H, Brendorp B, Pedersen OD, Kober L, Torp-Petersen C. Dofetilide: a new drug to control cardiac arrhythmia. *Expert Opin. Pharmacother.* 2003;**4**:973–985.

Saxonhouse SJ, Curtis AB. Risks and benefits of rate control versus maintenance of sinus rhythm. *Am. J. Cardiol.* 2003;**91**:27D–32D.

Sosin MD, Bhatia GS, Lip GYH. Should heart failure be treated with antithrombotic drugs? *Heart Drug* 2002;**2**:295–302.

Table 42 Drugs interacting with warfarin

Increased risk of bleeding
- Analgesics – aspirin, azapropazone
- Antiarrythmics – amiodarone, propafenone
- Antibiotics – ciprofloxacin, erythromycin, clarithromycin, metronidazole, fluconazole, itraconazole, ketoconazole
- Antidepressants – SSRIs
- Antiepileptics – valproate, phenytoin
- Cytotoxics – ifosfamide, fluorouracil
- Lipid-lowering drugs – fibrates and statins
- Thyroxine
- Ulcer-healing drugs – cimetidine, omeprazole

Decreased anticoagulant effect
- Antibiotics – rifampicin (rifampin), griseofulvin
- Antidepressants – St John's wort
- Antiepileptics – carbamazepine, primidone, phenytoin
- Cytotoxics – azathioprine
- Oral contraceptives

SSRI: selective serotonin reuptake inhibitor.

Chapter nine

Nonpharmacological therapies for heart failure

Introduction

Despite advances in medical therapy for heart failure (HF), mortality has remained depressingly high. Many patients with comorbidities are additionally unable to tolerate optimal drug therapy. A wide variety of nonpharmacological approaches is available to complement pharmacologic therapy in HF, ranging from simple education to costly and technologically advanced implantable devices. This chapter will discuss the place of these various therapies in the management of HF.

Education

Patients and relatives may benefit directly from education concerning the condition, providing realistic expectations for the future, and strategies for coping with symptoms. In addition, patients who understand their condition are more likely to comply with medication (*Table 43*). Patients may be taught about the need for regular stepwise increases in medication, and warning signs such as increasing breathlessness or oedema which suggest the need for urgent review. Mobile patients may be able to

Table 43 Evidence for multidisciplinary interventions in heart failure

Outcome	Result
Mortality	No evidence available
Quality of life; functional capacity; patient satisfaction; compliance (diet, medication); patient knowledge	Improved in trials that reported these outcomes
Hospital readmission over 1–6 months	Conflicting results between 4 small and 1 larger RCTs

RCT	n	ART (%)	ARC (%)	ARR (%)	RRR (%)	NNT
4	543	31	45	14 (6–21)	31 (13–47)	7 (5–17)
1	504	52	42	-11 (-19– -2)	-26 (-46– -5)	-9 (-20– -2)

Harms	No evidence available

While there are problems with the available data (small studies, highly selected patients, in academic centres, interventions varied, study time <6 months) it is likely that such interventions are beneficial.

ARC: absolute risk in control group; ARR: absolute risk reduction; ART: absolute risk in treatment group; NNT: number needed to treat; RCT: randomized controlled trial; RRR: relative risk reduction.

monitor their own weight at home, and possibly to vary the dose of their diuretics accordingly. Support from a specialist HF clinic, which may be led by appropriately trained nursing staff, can be invaluable (232). One study (Rich *et al.*, 1995) found that a multi-disciplinary approach with assessment by a geriatric cardiologist and intensive nurse education and support (dietary, social services, telephone contact) in a group of 282 patients resulted in fewer rehospitalizations, a trend towards extended survival, and lower healthcare costs compared with conventional therapy (*Table 44*).

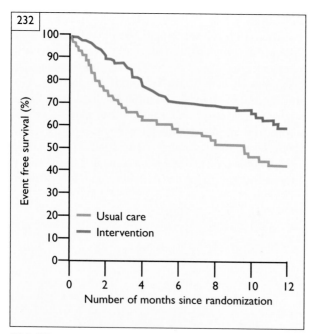

232 Effect of specialist nurse intervention on all-cause mortality/readmission in heart failure. Specialist intervention reduced endpoints (p=0.033). (From Blue L, *et al. BMJ* 2001;**323**:715–718.)

LIFESTYLE

As well as being involved in the development of coronary artery disease and thus development and progression of HF, smoking may result in tachycardia and increased systemic and pulmonary vascular resistance and blood pressure, and thus may further impair cardiac performance. All patients with HF, irrespective of aetiology, should therefore be encouraged to stop smoking.

High alcohol intake may predispose to arrythmias, as well as exerting a direct depressant effect on the myocardium. All patients with HF should therefore be advised to restrict alcohol intake to moderate levels. Patients with cardiomyopathy caused by alcohol should be advised to abstain completely; the prognosis is poor in patients who continue drinking or resume drinking after a period of abstinence.

Dietary advice is important; weight loss is beneficial in the obese both in terms of reducing cardiac work, and in reducing the risk of further cardiac events in ischaemic heart disease. Restriction of sodium and fluid intake may reduce peripheral oedema, although it has not been shown to reduce mortality in HF.

Patients with moderate to severe HF (NYHA class III or IV) have a high risk of morbidity and mortality with pregnancy, and therefore appropriate patients should receive counselling with regard to the optimal method of contraception.

IMMUNIZATION

Acute exacerbations of HF may be precipitated by intercurrent viral or bacterial infections. Patients with chronic HF should receive annual influenza vaccinations, and be considered for pneumococcal vaccination.

Table 44 Effect of multidisciplinary intervention on heart failure readmission (90 days) or death

	Control group (n=140)	Treatment group (n=142)	Reduction (%)
Readmisssion for decompensation	54	24	56.2
Readmission for other causes	40	29	28.5 (NS)
Hospital days per patient	6.2	3.9	36.6
Deaths	17	13	24.6 (NS)

Overall cost reduction per patient: $460

NS: nonsignificant. (From Rich MW, *et al. N. Engl. J. Med.* 1995;**333**:1190–1195.)

Table 45 Comparison between prescribed exercise and no prescribed exercise on cardiac events, mortality, and readmission in heart failure in a single randomized control trial (n = 99)

Outcome	ART(%)	ARC(%)	ARR(%)	RRR (%)	NNT
Cardiac event	34	76	42 (20–58)	55 (27–77)	2 (2–5)
Mortality	18	41	23 (5–41)	56 (13–80)	4 (2–20)
Readmission	10	29	19 (3–25)	65 (12–88)	6 (3–33)

Quality of life was improved (p<0.001), no evidence was reported about harms. ARC: absolute risk in control group; ARR: absolute risk reduction; ART: absolute risk in treatment group; NNT: number needed to treat; RRR: relative risk reduction.

ANTIBIOTICS

Patients with HF due to underlying primary valve disease require antibiotic prophylaxis prior to dental and other surgery.

Exercise

In previous years, patients with HF were advised to take bed rest, particularly during acute exacerbations. While patients with more severe symptomatic HF may need to avoid strenuous exertion, complete lack of exercise leads to atrophy of skeletal muscle and decreased functional capacity, and should not be encouraged. Indeed, a programme of exercise training may be beneficial to patients with HF, similar to postmyocardial infarction patients. Exercise training in patients with NYHA class II–III HF has been shown to have beneficial effects on exercise capacity, cytokine expression, heart rate variability, and endothelial function although there are no convincing data showing improvement in mortality (*Table 45*).

Devices for support during acute decompensation

Patients with acutely decompensated HF often present in extremis, and may deteriorate rapidly despite appropriate pharmacological therapy. These patients should be considered for some form of ventilatory or circulatory support to provide time for pharmacologic treatments to work, or as a bridge to definitive surgical management.

ASSISTED VENTILATION

Noninvasive ventilation

Noninvasive ventilation (NIV) is a form of ventilatory support which does not require paralysis and intubation. Positive pressure is provided via a tight fitting face or nasal mask (**233**). Continuous positive airways pressure (CPAP) has an accepted role in the treatment of sleep apnoea syndromes. Recently it has been recognized that sleep apnoea is

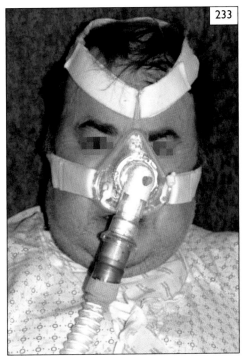

233 Patient with an exacerbation of chronic heart failure with noninvasive ventilatory support via a tight fitting nasal mask.

prevalent in HF, and may play a role in its development and progression. In addition, NIV has favourable effects on intrathoracic and left ventricular (LV) transmural pressures in patients with congestive HF. NIV has been used to treat acute HF. Several randomized trials have suggested that the use of CPAP results in more rapid increase in PaO_2, decrease in PCO_2, and lower rates of intubation compared to standard treatment. NIV may be considered in patients with rising PCO_2 levels despite adequate medical therapy. To be used successfully, NIV requires careful attention to mask fitting, and close patient observation. NIV should be used only in a high dependency setting, with appropriately trained staff. Some patients are not able to tolerate the necessary tight fitting mask, or may find the positive pressure 'suffocating'. In addition, due to changes in intrathoracic pressure, NIV may result in decreased blood pressure, limiting its usefulness in hypotensive HF patients.

Intermittent positive pressure ventilation
Patients with evidence of exhaustion or worsening arterial blood gases despite adequate treatment should be considered for invasive ventilation. The prognosis of patients with such refractory pulmonary oedema is poor, but some patients may show dramatic improvement after only a short period of intermittent positive pressure ventilation (IPPV). IPPV results in decreased venous return due to increased intrathoracic pressure, and therefore can have a deleterious effect upon blood pressure. Blood pressure must be maintained (with inotropic agents if necessary) before intubation. Input from the multidisciplinary team including cardiology, anaesthetics, and the patient or relatives should be sought when deciding whether to proceed to intubation.

INTRAAORTIC BALLOON COUNTERPULSATION
Intraaortic balloon counterpulsation (IABP) is an invasive strategy to preserve coronary flow in the presence of very poor cardiac output. A percutaneous approach is used to position a balloon in the descending aorta. The balloon is inflated during diastole, resulting in increased cardiac perfusion. This technique may be used to maintain circulation to the heart and brain as a bridge to transplantation or other definitive surgical intervention (234, 235).

Devices for long-term support of the failing ventricle

Due to the limited supply of transplant hearts, devices have been developed to attempt to support the failing heart, and to optimize efficiency of the remaining contractility. Such devices are becoming widely available, although costs remain high.

LEFT VENTRICULAR ASSIST DEVICE
A variety of surgically implanted devices have been developed to provide support to the failing LV, termed left ventricular assist devices (LVADs). Commonly, an inflow cannula receives blood from the LV, which is then pumped out through a cannula in the ascending aorta. Although initially used as a bridge to transplantation, some studies have demonstrated recovery of function allowing explantation of the device after a period of LV support, in certain subgroups of patients. Choice of LVAD will depend upon availability and local expertise.

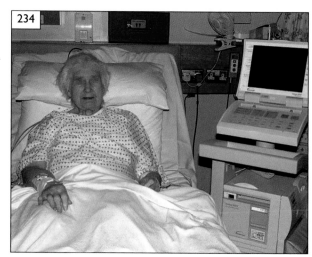

234 Patient on transfemoral intraaortic balloon pump support.

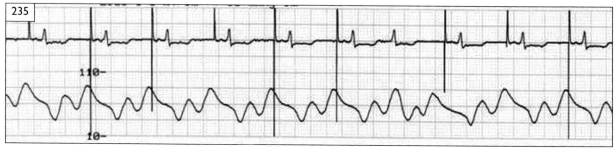

235 Intraaortic balloon pump monitoring showing electrocardiogram (upper trace) and intraaortic pressure trace (lower trace).

The main complications of LVADs include thromboembolism, right ventricular failure, and device failure (equivalent to severe aortic regurgitation, as the devices do not have valves). Careful patient selection is necessary to gain most benefit from such devices.

CARDIAC RESYNCHRONIZATION THERAPY
Patients with HF may exhibit dysynchronous contraction of the LV, resulting from abnormal electrical conduction pathways. Typically this results in septal contraction occurring some time before contraction of the free wall of the LV. Such dyssynchronous contraction results in significant circulation of blood in the LV cavity, rather than forward flow of blood. The use of biventricular pacing to restore synchronous contraction of the LV (cardiac resynchronization therapy, CRT) has increased in popularity in recent years. In addition to right ventricular and atrial pacing leads, a third lead is placed via the coronary sinus to pace the free wall of the LV (236, 237). However, the optimal method for selecting patients for CRT is not yet clear.

Present guidelines use duration of the electrocardiogram (ECG) QRS complex (*Table 46*); however, recent studies have shown that some patients with narrow QRS complexes may benefit from CRT and, equally, not all patients with wide QRS complexes benefit. Echocardiographic evidence of dyssynchronous contraction may prove to be a better method of selecting candidates for CRT.

In some patients, technical difficulties may preclude successful transvenous placement of the free wall pacing lead, in which case it may be placed epicardially through a limited thoracotomy.

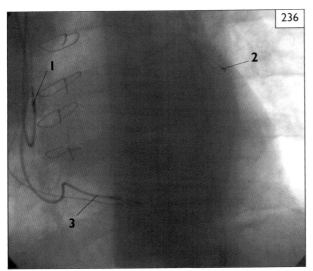

236 Fluoroscopic image following insertion of a biventricular pacemaker in a patient with previous coronary artery bypass grafting (note sternal wires). 1: right atrial lead; 2: left ventricular lead; 3: right ventricular lead. (Courtesy of Dr K. Patel.)

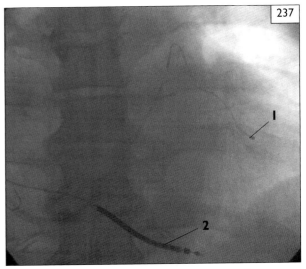

237 Fluoroscopic image following insertion of a combined biventricular pacemaker/defibrillator device. 1: left ventricular lead; 2: right ventricular pacing/defibrillation lead. (Courtesy of Dr K. Patel.)

Table 46 UK NICE recommendations for cardiac resynchronization therapy

CRT should be considered in selected patients with:
✧ LV systolic dysfunction (LVEF ≤35%)
✧ Drug refractory symptoms
✧ QRS duration >120 ms

The results of ongoing trials will help to guide appropriate patient selection. CRT: cardiac resynchronization therapy; LV: left ventricular; LVEF: left ventricular ejection fraction; NICE: National Institute for Clinical Excellence.

IMPLANTABLE CARDIOVERTER DEFIBRILLATOR

Patients with HF frequently suffer from sudden death. Although it is now recognized that some episodes of sudden death are caused by thrombosis such as pulmonary embolism, it is clear that malignant arrythmias are a common mode of death in HF. Surprisingly therefore, multiple trials of a variety of antiarrythmic drugs in HF have failed to show a mortality benefit. Routine use of antiarrythmic drugs in patients with HF is therefore not recommended. In contrast, recent studies involving the use of implantable cardioverter defibrillator (ICD) devices in patients with reduced ejection fraction following myocardial infarction (MI) have shown reduced mortality. However, the recent COMPANION study, which compared optimal medical treatment to optimal medical treatment plus cardiac resynchronization therapy with or without ICD therapy, did not find evidence of additional mortality benefit from ICD. The recent SCD-HeFT trial of ICD implantation involving >2500 patients with NYHA II–III showed a significant reduction in mortality at 5 years (hazard ratio 0.77), with greater benefit among those in NYHA II. However, routine ICD use in all patients would be prohibitively expensive in most countries. Further data to guide exactly which patients benefit from ICD are needed. Current UK NICE indications for ICD therapy in HF are listed in *Table 47*.

Interventional approaches

REVASCULARIZATION

In recent years, the phenomena of 'stunned' and 'hibernating' myocardium have been recognized and widely investigated. 'Hibernating' myocardium is defined as poorly functioning myocardium due to reduced perfusion, that may recover function if perfusion is restored. 'Stunned' myocardium results from an episode of ischaemia; the segment of myocardium regains normal blood flow after the episode, but recovery of function is delayed (although recovery occurs spontaneously). In patients with chronic ischaemic cardiomyopathy, revascularization (by either percutaneous intervention or coronary artery bypass grafting) may therefore result in improvement in LV function (**238, 239**).

Patients with cardiogenic shock due to acute MI have a very poor prognosis. Several restrospective studies suggested improved outcomes in cardiogenic

---

Table 47 UK NICE recommendations for implantable cardioverter defibrillators

ICD use should be routinely considered for patients in the following categories:

Secondary prevention, i.e. for patients who present, in the absence of a treatable cause with:

◇ Cardiac arrest due to either VT or VF

◇ Spontaneous sustained VT causing syncope or significant haemodynamic compromise

◇ Sustained VT without syncope/cardiac arrest and who have an associated reduction in EF (<35%) but are no worse than NYHA III*

Primary prevention for patients with:

◇ A history of previous MI and all of the following:

　◇ Nonsustained VT on Holter 24-hour ECG

　◇ Inducible VT on electrophysiological testing

◇ LV dysfunction with an EF <35% and are no worse than NYHA III*

◇ A familial cardiac condition with a high risk of sudden death including long QT syndrome, hypertrophic cardiomyopathy, Brugada syndrome, arrhythmogenic right ventricular dysplasia, and following repair of tetralogy of Fallot

◇ Marked limitation of physical activity. Although patients are comfortable at rest, less than ordinary physical activity will lead to symptoms (symptomatically moderate heart failure)

* Marked limitation of physical activity (moderate heart failure).

ECG: electrocardiogram; EF: ejection fraction; ICD: implantable cardioverter defibrillator; LV: left ventricular; MI: myocardial infarction; NICE: National Institute for Clinical Excellence; NYHA: New York Heart Association; VF: ventricular fibrillation; VT: ventricular tachycardia.

shock with revascularization. An analysis of outcomes of patients with cardiogenic shock in Israel showed improved survival in centres with facilities for acute intervention. The prospective SHOCK (SHould we emergently revascularize occluded coronaries for cardiogenic shOCK?) randomized patients to either conservative therapy (including thrombolysis and IABP where necessary), or invasive therapy with angiography and revascularization where appropriate. Although there was an 'early hazard' (excess mortality in the first 5 days in the intervention group) and mortality was not different at 30 days, 6- and 12-month follow-up, there was a significant survival advantage in the intervention group. Increasing availability of revascularization may improve survival in cardiogenic shock in the future.

VALVE REPLACEMENT/REPAIR

Patients with severe HF due to valvular heart disease, or functional mitral regurgitation, may benefit from valve replacement or repair (**240**). Ideally, surgery should be delayed until the patient is stable, but selected patients not improving on initial therapy may benefit from emergent valve replacement, although such patients are inherently high risk for such major surgery. A multidisciplinary team consisting of cardiologist, cardiovascular surgeon, and intensivist/anaesthetist will be needed to select suitable patients for intervention. A full discussion of indications for surgery is beyond the scope of this chapter.

238, 239 Percutaneous intervention (angioplasty) to the right coronary artery. **238**: Right coronary artery occluded proximally. **239**: Following the procedure, contrast passes down the right coronary artery.

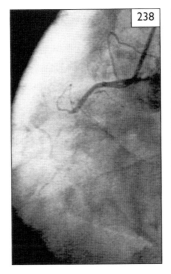
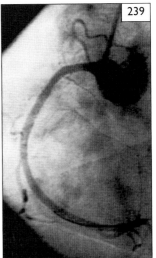

240 Mitral valvuloplasty. Inoue balloon is inflated across mitral valve. Patient has had previous cardiac surgery, note the sternal wires. 1: mitral valve; 2: inoue balloon.

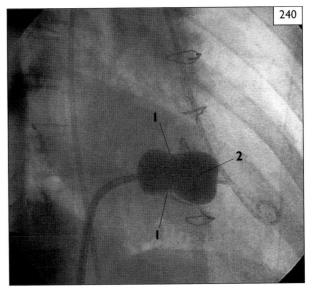

HEART TRANSPLANTATION

Patients with severe heart failure (NYHA IV) due to a nonreversible cause should be considered for heart transplantation, which remains the most effective therapy for end-stage heart failure (**241**). The number of available donor hearts is far short of the number of potential recipients: more than half of eligible patients die while awaiting transplantation. Despite efforts to increase the availability of donor hearts, many centres have noted a reduction in the number of procedures performed over recent years. The 10-year survival rate in cardiac transplantation now approaches 50% in carefully selected patients, with modern immunosupression regimens.

OTHER SURGICAL PROCEDURES

A number of alternative surgical procedures have been developed, due to the shortage of donor hearts for transplantation. LV reconstruction surgery (e.g. the Batista procedure), in which part of the LV is resected with the goal of increasing contractility, showed initial promise in patients with globally dilated, poorly functioning LV due to Chagas disease in South America. However, results have been inconsistent in patients with ischaemic cardiomyopathy, probably due to the patchy nature of the disease, and therefore these procedures are not performed widely.

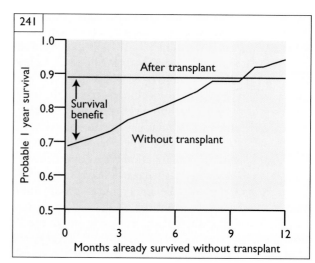

241 Relationship between survival on transplant waiting list (n=214) and survival after transplantation (n=88). Patients who survive >6–9 months on the waiting list appear to be at lower risk for death and therefore may derive less survival benefit from transplantation. (From Stevenson LW, et al. J. Am. Coll. Cardiol. 1991;**18**:919.)

Further reading

Bradley TD, Floras JS. Sleep apnea and heart failure. *Circulation* 2003;**107**:1671–1678.

Madani MM. Mitral valve repair in the treatment of heart failure. *Curr. Treat. Options Cardiovasc. Med.* 2004;**6**(4):305–311.

Mansfield DR, Gollogly NC, Kaye DM, Richardson M, Bergin P, Naughton MT. Controlled trial of continuous positive airway pressure in obstructive sleep apnoea and heart failure. *Am. J. Respir. Crit. Care Med.* 2004;**169**(3):361–366.

Nesser HJ, Breithardt OA, Khandheria BK. Established and evolving indications for cardiac resynchronization. *Heart* 2004;**90**(Suppl 6):vi 5–9.

Park SJ, Tector A, Piccioni W, et al. Left ventricular assist devices as destination therapy: a new look at survival. *J. Thorac. Cardiovasc. Surg.* 2005;**129**(1):9–17.

Paul S, Sneed NV. Strategies for behaviour change in patients with heart failure. *Am. J. Crit. Care* 2004;**13**(4):305–313.

Rich MW, Beckham V, Wittenberg C, et al. A multidisciplinary intervention to prevent the readmission of elderly patients with congestive heart failure. *N. Engl. J. Med.* 1995;**333**:1190–1195.

Sanborn TA, Feldman T. Management strategies for cardiogenic shock. *Curr. Opin. Cardiol.* 2004;**19**(6):608–612.

Chapter ten

Heart failure in primary care

Introduction

Although some patients with heart failure (HF) present acutely to the emergency department, many more develop the symptoms of HF insidiously, and so are more likely to present initially to their general practitioner (GP). HF is common, so every GP is likely to see such patients frequently. The GP therefore plays a vital role in the detection of HF. A GP with a list size of 2000 patients is likely to have around 25 patients with HF, and a future 25 with asymptomatic left ventricular (LV) dysfunction. Each year such a GP will see approximately 8–10 new possible diagnoses of HF, of which 3–4 will be confirmed. In addition, most patients with HF will need close supervision during titration of medications such as angiotensin-converting enzyme (ACE) inhibitors and β-blockers. Although this may well be under the supervision of a specialist HF clinic, such patients may well present to their GP if they suffer side-effects from these medications. Patients with HF also suffer frequent intercurrent illnesses, treatment of which may be complicated by, or themselves complicate HF symptoms or medications (*Table 48*). It is therefore important that all GPs are familiar with the diagnosis, monitoring, and treatment of HF.

Table 48 Major comorbidities that impact on the management of heart failure

Comorbidity	Comments
COPD/asthma/ reversible airways disease	β-blockers are contraindicated in patients with reversible airways disease. The British National Formulary (48th edn., 2004) states 'β-blockers should be avoided in patients with a history of asthma or chronic obstructive airways disease; if there is no alternative, a cardioselective β-blocker may be used with extreme caution under specialist supervision'.
Renal dysfunction (e.g. serum creatinine >200 μmol/l [2.3 mg/dl])	ACE inhibitors and angiotensin II receptor antagonists may be contraindicated. Patient requires specialist assessment
Anaemia	Anaemia is common in patients with moderate to severe heart failure and where due to heart failure (and not other causes) treatment with erythropoietin and iron therapy may improve symptoms and reduce the risk of hospitalization for worsening heart failure. The results of several large RCTs addressing this issue are awaited
Thyroid disease	Severe thyroid dysfunction may cause or precipitate heart failure
Peripheral vascular disease	Not an absolute contraindication to β-blocker therapy. High index of suspicion for renal artery stenosis required
Urinary frequency	Requires appropriate specialist referral. α-blockers may cause hypotension or fluid retention, but are not absolutely contraindicated in patients with heart failure. Diuretics likely to be less well tolerated
Gout	Avoid NSAIDs. Gout can be exacerbated by diuretics and may have an atypical presentation in patients with heart failure. Colchicine may be useful for the treatment of an acute attack of gout. Allopurinol may be useful at reducing the risk of further attacks of gout, but should not be started at the time of an acute episode of gout

ACE: angiotensin-converting enzyme; COPD: chronic obstructive pulmonary disease; NSAID: nonsteroidal anti-inflammatory drug; RCT: randomized controlled trial.

Management goals

As discussed earlier, HF is a disease with high rates of mortality and complications. The goals of therapy are to improve and maintain quality of life, including improved functional status. Extension of life is also a goal, but for many patients with advanced HF, this may be of secondary importance. The general practitioner may often be faced with decisions regarding medications which improve the patient's prognosis, but are associated with side-effects. Certainly where side-effects are causing impairment to the patient's quality of life, dose reduction may need to be considered, despite the reduction in mortality benefit that may occur.

Prevention

General practitioners have a vital role in the prevention of HF. Clearly, prevention is far superior to treatment, despite the many recent advances in HF therapy. Lifestyle advice such as smoking cessation and weight loss, appropriate lipid lowering therapy, and early recognition and treatment of angina may prevent myocardial infarction (MI) leading to HF. Rigorous control of blood pressure and diabetes is also central to the prevention of HF.

Accuracy of diagnosis

As HF tends to present with nonspecific symptoms, and often with few physical signs, a high index of suspicion is needed in patients with risk factors for HF, such as a history of ischaemic heart disease or hypertension. It is important to remember that dilated cardiomyopathy may occur at any age, and to consider this diagnosis in young breathless patients. Appropriate initial investigations would include chest X-ray, electrocardiogram (ECG), urea and electrolytes, thyroid function tests, and full blood count. If chest X-ray and ECG are entirely normal, HF is extremely unlikely. Patients in whom HF is suspected should ideally be referred for an objective assessment of myocardial function (most commonly echocardiography).

Studies which have used echocardiographic screening have found that patients with a diagnosis of 'heart failure' listed in their general practice records often do not actually have evidence of impairment of left ventricular function. The recent ECHOES (Echocardiographic heart of England Screening) study found that only 22% of patients listed as having HF by their GP actually had definite HF; a further 16% were found to have borderline HF. Similarly, prescription of diuretics has been shown to correspond poorly to the presence of definite HF. The emerging evidence of the importance of diastolic HF may further complicate the situation in general practice; echocardiographic criteria for the diagnosis of diastolic HF are controversial, and treatment is different from that of systolic HF.

Who to refer?

Although ideally all patients with suspected HF should be assessed by a cardiologist specializing in HF, the prevalence of the condition is such that this is unlikely to be a realistic goal. However, referral is certainly necessary where symptoms are severe, where the diagnosis is in doubt, where patients do not respond to therapy, or where there is suspicion of significant valve disease or other structural heart disease.

Access to echocardiography

OPEN ACCESS ECHOCARDIOGRAPHY

In many areas, GPs may refer direct for echocardiography, which may be beneficial to patients in reducing delay to diagnosis. However, GPs who are not themselves familiar with echocardiography may have difficulty interpreting echocardiography reports, particularly where the results are borderline.

SPECIALIST HEART FAILURE CLINICS

In some areas, cardiologists specializing in HF may have a specialist HF clinic, ideally supported by a specialist HF nurse (242). Referral to such a clinic may have advantages over open access echocardio-

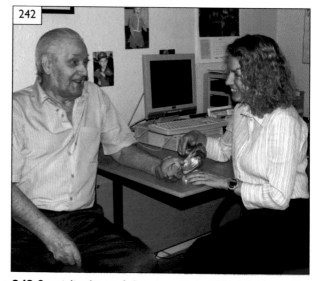

242 Specialist heart failure nurse consultation.

graphy in that the echocardiographic findings are interpreted by an HF specialist, rather than being returned to the GP for further action. In addition, the patient can receive education (*Table 49*), be immediately commenced on appropriate initial medication, and arrangements can be made for dose titration, without the need for a further referral from the GP.

PORTABLE ECHOCARDIOGRAPHY

Increasing availability of portable echocardiography machines may enable more GPs to have access to echocardiography in the community (Chambers *et al.*, 2004). Some GPs with previous experience may be able to use these machines themselves; others may require community technicians to perform scans. Some portable machines possess sufficient functionality to perform a full echocardiographic study, others are suitable only for a limited study, which may identify patients who require referral for full examination.

Screening for asymptomatic left ventricular dysfunction

The recognition that ACE inhibitors may delay or prevent progression from asymptomatic left ventricular dysfunction to HF has led to the suggestion of screening patients in the community. However, screening a large population with echocardiography is prohibitively expensive and time consuming. Additionally, since it is clear from studies (such as HOPE – Heart Outcomes Prevention Evaluation) that all patients with MI, as well as patients with diabetes plus one additional risk factor (such as smoking or hypertension) benefit from ACE inhibition whether or not they have LV dysfunction, it is not yet clear who should be screened. Brain natriuretic peptide (BNP) or NT-proBNP does not have sufficient positive predictive value to be used as a sole screening method, as it would generate many false-positive results (*Table 50*). Additionally, as it is raised in both systolic and diastolic dysfunction as well as atrial fibrillation (AF), even a true positive result would not be sufficient to start treatment with an ACE inhibitor. The best policy may be to screen patients at risk of HF, but who do not have other indications for ACE inhibition with BNP (or NT-proBNP), followed by echocardiography for those with an abnormal result.

Table 49 Topics for education and counselling in heart failure

General topics
✧ Explanation of heart failure
✧ Expected symptoms versus symptoms of worsening heart failure
✧ Psychological responses
✧ Prognosis

Management
✧ Self-monitoring measurement of weight weekly (daily if unstable)
✧ Action plan in case of increased symptoms
✧ Dietary recommendations
✧ Sodium restriction
✧ Fluid restriction
✧ Alcohol restriction

Activity level
✧ Activity and exercise
✧ Work and leisure activities
✧ Exercise programme
✧ Sexual activity

Compliance strategies
✧ Medication
✧ Nature of each drug, dosing, and side-effects
✧ Coping with a complicated regimen
✧ Cost issues

(From Grady KL, *et al. Circulation* 2000;**102**:2443.)

Table 50 Sensitivity and specificity of brain natriuretic peptides in the diagnosis of chronic heart failure

	New diagnosis of HF (primary care)	LV systolic dysfunction
Sensitivity (%)	97	77
Specificity (%)	84	87
+ve predictive value (%)	70	16

HF: heart failure; LV: left ventricular.
(From Cowie MR, *et al. Lancet* 1997;**350**:1349; McDonagh TA, *et al. Lancet* 1998;**351**:9–13.)

Nondrug management

General practitioners are likely to be more aware of a patient's long-term quality of life than hospital colleagues. There may be additional nondrug interventions which can improve quality of life significantly, which the GP is well placed to suggest to the patient. Occupational therapy assessment and provision of aids to enable patients with more severe HF to carry out activities of daily living may be helpful. Patients may find it difficult to manage complicated drug regimens; pharmacists may be able to help by providing weekly drug packs.

Drug treatment

DIURETICS

A trial of a loop diuretic may be worthwhile in patients with symptoms of HF, with improvement in symptoms providing some evidence towards a diagnosis of HF. Monitoring of renal function is advisable, particularly in patients on high doses of diuretics. It is important to consider dose reduction once patients are stabilized, as high-dose loop diuretics may, in the long term, lead to renal impairment and ototoxicity. Hypokalaemia is common with diuretics, particularly at high doses, or if combinations of loop and thiazide diuretics are used. Gout is also a common side-effect of diuretics, which can be difficult to manage as nonsteroidal anti-inflammatory drugs (NSAIDs) should be avoided in HF. Treatment should be with colchicine, followed by allopurinol once the acute episode has settled, together with diuretic dose reduction if possible.

ANGIOTENSIN-CONVERTING ENZYME INHIBITORS

ACE inhibitors are, in general, safe to initiate in the community. Where the suspicion of HF is high, it is reasonable to initiate treatment with an ACE inhibitor prior to referral for echocardiography. Monitoring of renal function is advisable before initiation of an ACE inhibitor, and 1–2 weeks after increasing the dose. It is important to note that a small rise in serum creatinine is normal with ACE inhibition. Patients who do not tolerate ACE inhibitors due to cough may be safely changed to an angiotensin-II receptor blocker, although monitoring of renal function is still necessary. Increasingly, patients are on combination treatment with spironolactone and an ACE inhibitor. Such a combination may lead to hyperkalaemia, which,

although rare in the setting of clinical trials, may be significant in the general HF population. Careful manipulation of each patient's prescription may be necessary to avoid hypo- or hyperkalaemia.

BETA-BLOCKERS

β-blockers were avoided in HF for many years due to their negative inotropic action. Rapid introduction of high doses of β-blockers may certainly lead to an episode of decompensation, but even with strict adherence to titration schedules, some patients may experience worsening of symptoms and may present to their GP. Dose reduction or withdrawal may be necessary. β-blockers may additionally cause fatigue, cold peripheries, erectile dysfunction, and nightmares; again if these are judged to impair quality of life significantly, dose reduction must be considered, despite the possible prognostic cost.

WARFARIN

Warfarin monitoring is frequently carried out under the supervision of GPs. With the advent of home testing monitors for the international normalized ratio (INR), it is likely that the monitoring of warfarin will become more community based. Patients with HF frequently take drugs which interact with warfarin, and may also have hepatic impairment, so represent a group at risk of bleeding from warfarin. Close observation of warfarin is essential, particularly at the time of introduction of other medications which may interact with warfarin.

DRUG COUNSELLING

Concordance with medication is poor among patients with any chronic disease. It is important to reinforce the importance of taking the prescribed medications regularly. The need for gradual dose titration of some medications may need careful explanation, and side-effects of drugs should be covered (e.g. ACE inhibitor-induced cough). Advice about what to do in special circumstances is important, e.g. inadvertently missing a dose of medication, or if intercurrent gastrointestinal infection occurs; in combination with diuretics this could lead to dehydration and diuretic dose may need to be reduced temporarily.

Specialist heart failure nurses

Increasingly, specialist HF nurses take the lead in patient monitoring and drug dose titration, with support from specialist consultants and GPs (**242**). Indeed, specialist nurses can provide a vital link between primary and secondary care. The specialist nurse is ideally placed to provide patient education, with reinforcement during regular assessments. Home visits by specialist nurses are invaluable to poorly mobile or breathless patients who may find it difficult to attend hospital for the regular appointments necessary during dose titration, or for monitoring of unstable patients (**243**). Early recognition of decompensation with early admission and intensive management, facilitated by specialist nurses, may lead to shorter hospital stays and improved overall quality of life. Indeed, studies of intensive interventions carried out in the United States and Australia, including specialist nurse visits and assessment by other health professionals, have shown marked reduction in admissions and length of stay at only a modest cost (offset by the reduced cost from reduced admissions).

Recommendations in the UK National Institute for Clinical Excellence (NICE) guidelines for assessments to be made during clinical review are summarized in *Table 51*.

Frequency of review

For patients who are clinically stable, 3–6 monthly review is recommended. Unstable patients may well need more frequent review by the GP or HF specialist nurse and, possibly, review by a cardiologist.

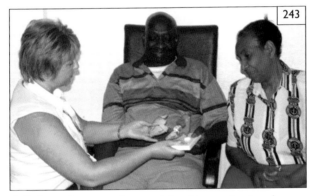

243 Specialist nurse home visit with a patient and his wife.

Table 51 Assessments to be made at clinical review	
Functional capacity	Chiefly from the history, but more objectively by use of NYHA class, specific quality of life questionnaires, 6-minute walk test, or maximal exercise test. Note: Not all of these tests are likely to be necessary or appropriate at each assessment
Fluid status	Chiefly by physical examination: changes in body weight, extent of jugular venous distension, lung crackles, hepatomegaly, extent of peripheral oedema, and lying and standing BP (postural drop in BP may indicate hypovolaemia)
Cardiac rhythm	Chiefly by clinical examination, but may require 12-lead ECG or 24-hour ECG Holter monitoring if suspicion of arrhythmia
Laboratory assessment	Checking of serum biochemistry (urea, electrolytes, creatinine) is essential, but other tests (such as thyroid function, haematology, liver function, level of anticoagulation) may also be required depending on the medication prescribed and comorbidity
BP: blood pressure; ECG: electrocardiogram; NYHA: New York Heart Association.	

Audit

Regular audit is a cornerstone of clinical governance. Studies suggest that many patients with HF are not prescribed ACE inhibitors and other evidence-based therapies. In the UK, the new contract for GPs included points for the establishment of a HF register, for newly diagnosed patients having undergone echocardiography, and for a high proportion of HF patients being prescribed ACE inhibitors. For all of these reasons, audit of HF patients within a GP list is important.

In England and Wales, the National Service Framework for Coronary Heart Disease suggests an annual audit of the care provided for patients with HF (*Table 52*).

In Scotland, a set of audit criteria has been suggested for patients with HF due to ischaemic heart disease (*Table 53*).

Table 52 National Service framework for coronary heart disease suggested audit topics

- ✧ Number and percentage of the registered population with a diagnosis of HF
- ✧ Number and percentage of patients with confirmed HF or LV dysfunction currently prescribed an ACE inhibitor
- ✧ Number and percentage of patients with a diagnosis of HF who have ever undergone echocardiography by practice and PCG/PCT
- ✧ Age/sex standardized admission rates for HF by PCG/PCT and Health Authority
- ✧ Age/sex standardized mortality rates for patients with HF/LV dysfunction
- ✧ Number and percentage of patients with HF for whom specialist palliative care advice has been sought by practice and PCG/PCT

ACE: angiotensin-converting enzyme; HF: heart failure; LV: left ventricular; PCG: Primary Care Group; PCT: Primary Care Trust

---

Table 53 Scottish programme for improving clinical effectiveness in primary care audit criteria

- ✧ Practices will have a database that records cardiac failure; there will be a system in place for adding new patients to the database and the detection of defaulters from follow-up
- ✧ Patients with newly suspected HF will have a 12-lead ECG performed
- ✧ Patients with newly suspected HF will have an echocardiogram if the ECG is abnormal; patients with existing clinically diagnosed HF will have had an echocardiogram at some time if possible
- ✧ Patients with suspected HF will have FBC, biochemical profile (urea and electrolytes, liver function tests), blood glucose, thyroid function test, and cholesterol evaluation
- ✧ Patients with suspected HF will have a medication review at diagnosis (including drugs known to worsen HF)
- ✧ Patients with HF will be treated with an ACE inhibitor unless contraindicated or unless there are significant side-effects
- ✧ Patients on ACE inhibitors for HF will be stabilized on recommended therapeutic doses
- ✧ Patients with HF will be prescribed a duiretic if there are symptoms or signs of fluid retention
- ✧ Patients with HF will be reviewed annually at a minimum, by an appropriately trained member of the primary care team; areas to be covered include clinical status and medication review
- ✧ Patients with HF will have their biochemistry checked at a minimum every year
- ✧ Patients with HF will receive an annual influenza vaccine unless there is specific contraindication
- ✧ Patients with HF will receive a one-off pneumococcal vaccine unless there is specific contraindication
- ✧ Patients who smoke tobacco should be advised and offered support to stop

ACE: angiotensin-converting enzyme; ECG: electrocardiogram; FBC: full blood count; HF: heart failure.

Further reading

Chambers J, Faut A, Liddiard S, *et al*. Community echocardiography for heart failure. *Br. J. Cardiol.* 2004;**11**(5):399–402.

Davis RC, Hobbs FD, Kenkre JE, *et al*. Prevalence of left ventricular systolic dysfunction and heart failure in high risk patients: community based epidemiological study. *BMJ* 2002;**325**:1156–1160.

Duffy JR, Hoskins LM, Chen MC. Nonpharmacological strategies for improving heart failure outcomes in the community: a systematic review. *J. Nurs. Care Qual.* 2004;**19**(4):349–360.

Khunti K, Hearnshaw H, Baker R, Grimshaw G. Heart failure in primary care: qualitative study of current management and perceived obstacles to evidence-based diagnosis and management by general practitioners. *Eur. J. Heart Fail.* 2002;**4**:771–777.

Lee WC, Chavez YE, Baker T, Luce BR. Economic burden of heart failure: a summary of recent literature. *Heart Lung* 2004;**33**(6):362–371.

Stewart S, Horowitz JD. Specialist nurse management programmes: economic benefits in the management of heart failure. *Pharmacoeconomics* 2003;**21**:225–240.

Stewart S, Jenkins A, Buchan S, McGuire A, Capewell S, McMurray JJ. The current cost of heart failure to the National Health Service in the UK. *Eur. J. Heart Fail.* 2002;**4**:361–371.

Stromberg A, Martensson J, Fridlund B, Levin LA, Karlsson JE, Dahlstrom U. Nurse-led heart failure clinics improve survival and self-care behaviour in patients with heart failure. Results from a prospective, randomized trial. *Eur. Heart J.* 2003;**24**:1014–1023.

Wang TJ, Levy D, Benjamin EJ, Vasan RS. The epidemiology of 'asymptomatic' left ventricular systolic dysfunction: implications for screening. *Ann. Intern. Med.* 2003;**138**:907–916.

Zile MR, Brutsaert DL. New concepts in diastolic dysfunction and diastolic heart failure: Part I: diagnosis, prognosis, and measurements of diastolic function. *Circulation* 2002;**105**:1387–1393.

Chapter eleven

The future of heart failure management

Introduction

As the burden of heart failure (HF) increases, so the search for new treatment options has increased. In this section, a number of novel medical and surgical approaches to the management of HF are described, that are currently at various stages of development.

Impedance cardiography

Impedance cardiography, or thoracic bioimpedance, is a form of plethysmography that uses changes in thoracic electrical impedance to estimate haemo-dynamic parameters such as cardiac output and thoracic fluid content (**244**). Some studies have suggested that the use of impedance cardiography in combination with assessment of brain natriuretic peptide (BNP) might aid diagnosis of HF in the emergency setting. More recently, implantable impedance monitors (combined with pacemaker defibrillator devices) have been developed, with the aim of early detection of impending decompensation by measuring trends in thoracic fluid content, with a view to prevention of the development of clinical decompensation and hospital admission. Large scale trials will be necessary to determine if such devices can prevent admissions and improve quality of life in patients with advanced HF.

Medical treatments

SILDENAFIL

Sildenafil, an inhibitor of phosphodiesterase-5A, results in accumulation of cyclic guanosine monophosphate (GMP), and is a widely used treatment for impotence. A recent study has demonstrated in a mouse model that sildenafil reduces the development of cardiac hypertrophy induced by banding the aorta compared to controls. In a further experiment, mice allowed to develop cardiac hypertrophy and then commenced on sildenafil were found to show regression of cardiac hypertrophy, whereas control mice showed continued hypertrophy. Clearly, further study is necessary before any conclusions can be drawn about the use of sildenafil in humans with cardiac hypertrophy or HF, but these early results are encouraging. Of note, sildenafil is contraindicated in patients taking nitrates; therefore, this treatment is unlikely to benefit patients with ischaemic cardiomyopathy.

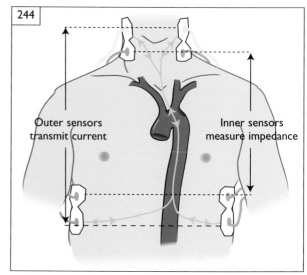

244 The noninvasive impedance cardiography monitor involves four pairs of electrodes positioned as shown. An alternating current is applied between pairs of electrodes, and the voltage measured constantly. As the current is constant, thoracic impedance can be calculated directly from changes in voltage, according to Ohm's law. A number of haemodynamic parameters can be estimated from the thoracic impedance.

STEM CELL THERAPY

For some years researchers have been studying the possibility of replacing poorly functioning or infarcted areas of myocardium with fresh cells, and thus improving cardiac contractility. A variety of cell types have been used, including skeletal myoblasts, fetal cardiomyocytes, and endothelial progenitor cells. However, recent research has focused on the use of pluripotent stem cells, which have the potential to differentiate fully into cardiomyocytes (unlike skeletal myoblasts and endothelial progenitor cells; the latter are in fact more likely to result in revascularization than direct improvement in contractile function). The use of embryonic stem cells is largely prevented currently by ethical and political barriers, and therefore attention has switched to the possibility of using bone marrow stromal cells harvested from adults. In particular, these cells can be harvested from the intended recipient, expanded in tissue culture, then returned (a so-called autologous procedure), avoiding the possibility of rejection by the patient's immune system. Unresolved issues with the use of stem cell therapy include the optimal mode of delivery (intravenous, direct intracardiac injection, or intracoronary delivery), and the high frequency of ventricular arrhythmia in recipients. The randomized Bone Marrow Transfer to Enhance ST-Elevation Infarct Regeneration Trial (BOOST) of intracoronary delivery of adult bone marrow stromal cells during percutaneous intervention has shown a significant benefit in terms of ejection fraction (EF) in patients receiving the cell replacement therapy (**245**) Available data suggest that this therapy may be beneficial in HF, but more robust studies with larger numbers and longer follow-up are required.

ERYTHROPOIETIN AND INTRAVENOUS IRON

Anaemia (haemoglobin <12 g/dl [120 g/l]) may be found in up to one-third of patients with HF, and is an independent risk factor for rehospitalization and mortality. Anaemia may occur due to chronic renal ischaemia, resulting in reduced production of erythropoietin by the kidney. Alternative theories include the possibility that inflammatory mediators such as interleukin-6 and tumour necrosis factor may interfere with the action of erythropoietin. Small studies suggest that correction of anaemia with subcutaneous erythropoietin and intravenous iron results in improved quality of life, reduced left ventricular (LV) mass, increased exercise tolerance, and reduced frequency of hospitalization, and may possibly slow the progression of HF. More recent data suggest that erythropoietin may inhibit apoptosis, preserve cellular membranes, and prevent inflammation, implying that erythropoietin may have additional benefit in HF besides correction of anaemia.

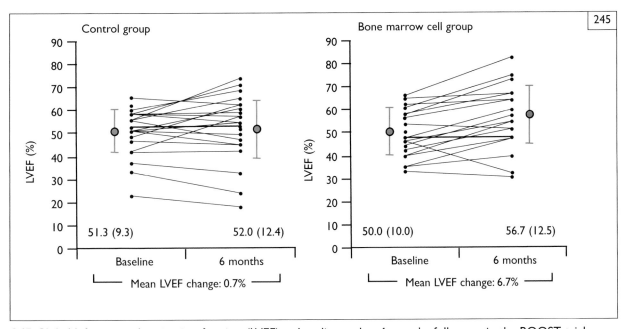

245 Global left ventricular ejection fraction (LVEF) at baseline and at 6 months follow-up in the BOOST trial.

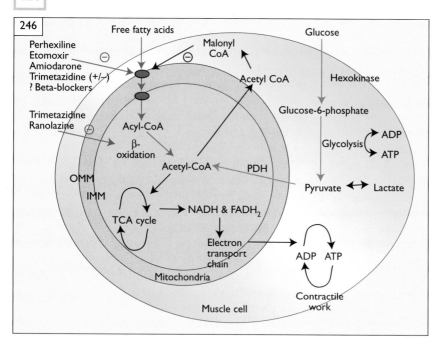

246 Diagram to show myocardial metabolism and sites of drug action. CPT, carnitine-palmitoyl-transferase; IMM, inner mitochondrial membrane; OMM, outer mitochondrial membrane; PDH, pyruvate dehydrogenase. Free-fatty-acid oxidative pathway in red. Glucose oxidative pathway in blue. From *Eur Heart J.* 2004 Apr;**25**(8):634-41.

METABOLIC TREATMENTS

A number of antianginal drugs that work by altering myocardial metabolism, with little effect on haemodynamics, have been available for some years. More recently, it has been suggested that these drugs may benefit patients with chronic HF. Examples of such drugs include perhexiline, ranolazine, etomoxir, and trimetazidine (**246**). These drugs act by switching the main energy source of myocardial tissue from free fatty acids to glucose, effectively reverting to the situation found in the fetal heart.

Metabolism of glucose requires less oxygen than that of free fatty acids to generate the same amount of energy, thus reducing myocardial oxygen demand. Small studies have suggested that such drugs may be associated with improvements in exercise tolerance and quality of life. Long-term data concerning safety and efficacy are currently lacking. Hepatotoxicity is a risk with perhexilene, and plasma monitoring is required to prevent this. Of note, recent studies have suggested that beta-blockers may achieve some of their benefits through similar metabolic effects.

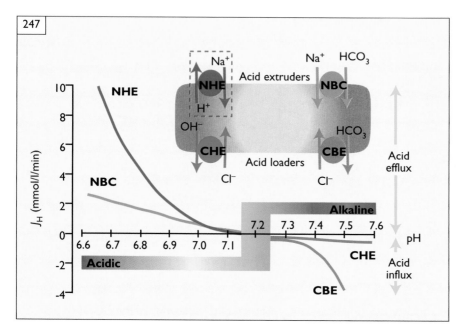

247 Diagram to show intracellular pH regulation. NHE-1 is one of four membrane proteins that are involved in pH regulation. Two of these are acid loaders, chloride hydroxyl exchanger (CHE) and chloride bicarbonate exchanger (CBE); the other two are acid extruders, sodium bicarbonates importer (NBC) and Na+/H+ exchanger (NHE). This graph shows pH on the x axis and proton flux on the y axis. (Adapted from Leem *et al. J. Physiol.* 1999;**517**:159–180.)

INHIBITION OF SODIUM–HYDROGEN EXCHANGE

The sodium–hydrogen exchange system is a ubiquitous membrane protein involved in pH regulation (247). During ischaemia, the cell becomes acidic, resulting in activation of the sodium–hydrogen exchanger. Hydrogen ions are exchanged for sodium, leading to a buildup of sodium within the cell. Inhibitors of this exchange pathway, such as the orally active drugs amiloride and cariporide, have been used in ischaemic heart disease, and are thought to act by reducing the influx of sodium into ischaemic myocardial cells. This is beneficial because intracellular sodium is re-exchanged for calcium, leading to accumulation of calcium within myocytes, which is thought to be an early step in myocardial necrosis. Sodium–hydrogen exchange inhibition may have other beneficial effects, such as reducing oxidative stress. Given early to patients with acute myocardial infarction (MI) in conjunction with reperfusion, cariporide may reduce infarct size. The Sodium–Proton Exchange Inhibition to Prevent Coronary Events in Acute Cardiac Conditions Trial (EXPEDITION) found that cariporide given intravenously at the time of surgery reduced nonfatal MI following coronary artery bypass, but was unfortunately associated with increased mortality (248, 249), apparently due to an increased risk of stroke, the mechanism of which was unclear.

By a similar mechanism it is possible that cariporide may prevent progression of HF. In a rabbit model, cariporide prevented the development of HF in rabbits subjected to volume and pressure overload. Further data are needed to assess the mechanism of increased stroke in the EXPEDITION trial, and whether this drug could be used safely in HF.

Surgical treatments

ANTIREMODELLING DEVICES

A number of devices designed to reverse or prevent cardiac remodelling are presently in development. The Myosplint device (Myocor, MN) is implanted surgically without the need for cardiopulmonary bypass. Three Myosplints are inserted, each consisting of two pads which rest on the outer surface of the heart connected by a cord passing through the LV perpendicular to the ventricular long axis (250). Once placed, the Myosplints draw the ventricular walls inward, creating a symmetric, bilobular LV. The safety and feasibility of the procedure has been confirmed in animal studies, and early human studies are now in progress.

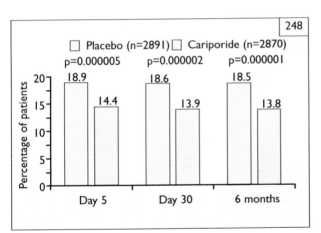

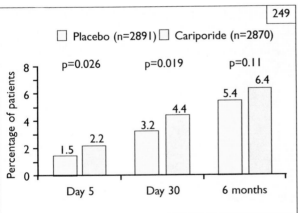

248, 249 Results from the EXPEDITION trial at 6 months follow-up. 248: Nonfatal myocardial infarction; 249: mortality.

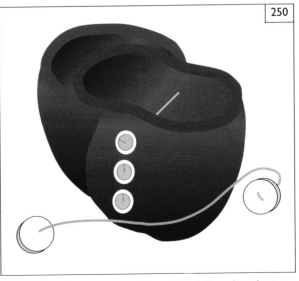

250 Schematic representation of the Myosplint device.

Another device currently in development is the CorCap Cardiac Support device (Acorn Cardio-vascular, MN), a synthetic mesh which surrounds the heart to prevent dilatation (**251**). The ACORN-CSD trial consisted of 300 patients, randomized to receive the CSD or standard therapy (in 193 cases the patients also underwent mitral valve surgery). CSD-treated patients showed reduction in LV volume and a reduction in major cardiac procedures such as transplantation. This encouraging preliminary data requires confirmation in further studies.

Treatment of functional mitral regurgitation

Open surgery for functional mitral regurgitation may be carried out at the time of coronary artery bypass surgery. The Coapsys system (Myocor, MN) works upon the same principle as the Myosplint, discussed above, using a system of cords to bring the mitral valve leaflets into apposition (**252**), and can be performed during off-pump coronary artery bypass surgery (i.e. surgery performed without cardio-pulmonary bypass, on the beating heart). This device is currently being assessed prospectively versus standard therapy in the randomized RESTOR-MV trial (Randomized Evaluation of Surgical Treatment for Off-pump Repair of the Mitral Valve).

Minimal access techniques are also being developed to correct functional mitral regurgitation, including the use of robotic-assisted laparoscopic systems such as the da Vinci system (Intuitive Surgical). These techniques offer the advantage of avoiding a sternotomy, but still require cardiopulmonary bypass. Long-term follow-up data will be needed to compare such new techniques to open surgery.

The total artificial heart

The mismatch between demand for heart transplantation and supply of donor hearts has led to the search for an alternative, a total artificial heart. The first such device, the AbioCor (Abiomed, Massachusetts) was unveiled in 2001 (**253, 254**). This device makes use of advances in energy transfer allowing it to be entirely implantable with no exteriorized wiring and, therefore, less chance of infection. To date, 10 patients have received an AbioCor implant, all of whom had an expected survival of <30 days. The longest survival following implantation is currently 512 days. The size of the device limits its suitability to only half of men and one-fifth of women. Clinical trials are ongoing. Another device, the CardioWest total artificial heart (**255**) (SynCardia, Arizona) has also been developed, and is currently indicated in patients with dilated cardiomyopathy as a bridge to transplantation. This device has been shown to improve the rate of survival to transplantation in such patients. The CardioWest is not totally implantable, requiring an external power source.

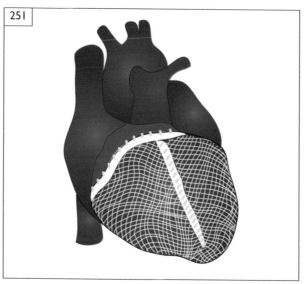

251 Diagram of the CorCap Cardiac Support device.

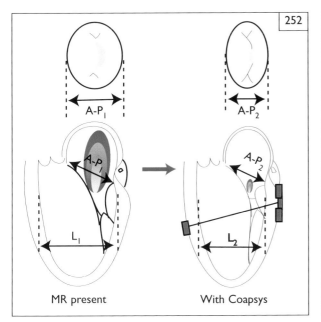

252 Diagramatic representation of the effect of the Coapsys system. MR: mitral regurgitation.

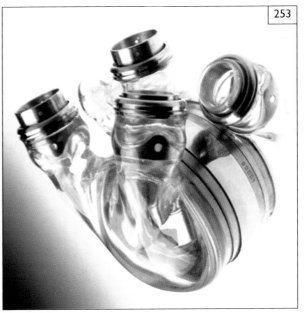

253 The AbioCor total artificial heart. (Courtesy of Abiomed Inc., Massachusetts, USA.)

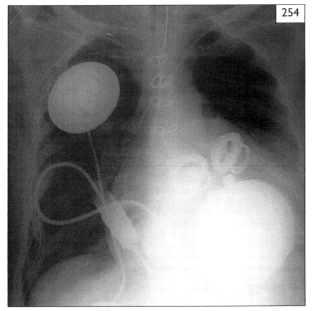

254 Chest X-ray of a patient after implantation of an AbioCor total artificial heart.

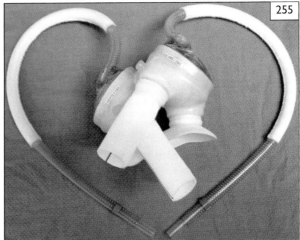

255 The CardioWest total artifical heart. (Courtesy of SynCardia Systems Inc., Arizona, USA.)

The future

HF is increasing in prevalence, and is likely to continue to do so as survival from conditions which predispose to HF (such as MI) increases. It is likely that HF will take up a larger proportion of both general practitioner and physician workload. HF is a huge economic burden (*Table 54*). The cost of HF in the UK has increased dramatically from approximately £360 million in 1993 to more than £900 million in 2000. Approximately 200 000 admissions each year occur as a result of HF and represent the majority of the cost of HF (*Table 55*). Prevention of HF, and prevention of episodes of decompensation in established HF are therefore very important healthcare goals in the future. Further research is essential to attempt to answer outstanding questions in the field of HF, such as the effect of ethnicity, the importance of diastolic HF, and the utility of screening for asymptomatic left ventricular dysfunction.

Table 54 Cost of heart failure

Country	Cost	% Healthcare costs	% Costs due to admissions
UK 1990–1991	£360m	1.2	60
USA 1989	$9bn	1.5	71
France 1990	FF11.4bn	1.9	64
New Zealand 1990	NZ$73m	1.5	68
Sweden 1990	Kr2.6m	2.0	75

(From McMurray J, et al. Br. J. Med. Econ. 1993;**6**:99–110.)

Table 55 Economic cost of heart failure to the NHS in the UK 1990–1991

	Total cost (£m)	%Total cost
GP visits	8.3	2.5
Referrals to hospital from GP	8.2	2.4
Inpatient stay	213.8	63.5
Diagnostic tests	45.6	13.5
Drugs	22.1	6.6

GP: general practitioner. (From McMurray J, et al. Br. J. Med. Econ. 1993;**6**:99–110. Selected data only presented.)

Further reading

Barcarse E, Kazanegra R, Chen A, Chiu A, Clopton P, Maisel A. Combination of B-type natriuretic peptide levels and noninvasive haemodynamic parameters in diagnosing congestive heart failure in the emergency department. *Congest. Heart Fail.* 2004;**10**(4):171–176.

Davani S, Deschaseaux F, Chalmers D, Tiberghien P, Kantelip JP. Can stem cells mend a broken heart? *Cardiovasc. Res.* 2005;**65**(2):305–316.

Lee L, Horowitz J, Frenneaux M. Metabolic manipulation in ischaemic heart disease, a novel approach to treatment. *Eur. Heart J.* 2004;**25**(8):634–641.

Maiese K, Li F, Chong ZZ. New avenues of exploration for erythropoietin. *J.A.M.A.* 2005;**293**(1):90–95.

Mentzer RM Jr, EXPEDITION Sodium–Proton Exchange Inhibition to Prevent Coronary Events in Acute Cardiac Conditions Trial. Abstract presentation at American Heart Association Scientific Sessions 2003.

Sabbah HN. The cardiac support device and the myosplint: treating heart failure by targeting left ventricular size and shape. *Ann. Thorac. Surg.* 2003;**75**(6):S13–19.

Samuels LE, Dowling R. Total artificial heart: destination therapy. *Cardiol. Clin.* 2003;**21**:115–118.

Silverberg DS, Wexler D, Iaina A. The role of anaemia in the progression of congestive heart failure. Is there a place for erythropoietin and intravenous iron? *J. Nephrol.* 2004;**17**(6):749–761.

Takimoto E, Champion HC, Li M, et al. Chronic inhibition of cyclic GMP phosphodiesterase-5A prevents and reverses cardiac hypertrophy. *Nature Med.* 2005;**11**(2):214–222.

Tatooles AJ, Pappas PS, Gordon PJ, Slaughter MS. Minimally invasive mitral valve repair using the da Vinci robotic system. *Ann. Thorac. Surg.* 2004;**77**(6):1978–1982.

Appendices

APPENDIX A
SEMINAL TRIALS

AHeFT: African-American Heart Failure Trial. (Study design)
Franciosa JA, Taylor AL, Cohn JN, *et al*. A-HeFT Investigators. African-American Heart Failure Trial (A-HeFT): rationale, design, and methodology. *J. Card. Fail.* 2002; 8(3):128–135.

AIRE: Acute Infarction Ramipril Efficacy Study.
The Acute Infarction Ramipril Efficacy (AIRE) Study Investigators. Effect of ramipril on mortality and morbidity of survivors of acute myocardial infarction with clinical evidence of heart failure. *Lancet* 1993;**342**(8875):821–828.

ATLAS: Assessment of Treatment with Lisinopril and Survival Trial.
Packer M, Poole-Wilson PA, Armstrong PW, *et al*. Comparative effects of low and high doses of the angiotensin-converting enzyme inhibitor, lisinopril, on morbidity and mortality in chronic heart failure. ATLAS Study Group. *Circulation* 1999;**100**(23):2312–2318.

BEST: Beta-blocker Evaluation Survival Trial.
Beta-Blocker Evaluation of Survival Trial Investigators. A trial of the beta-blocker bucindolol in patients with advanced chronic heart failure. *N. Engl. J. Med.* 2001;**344**(22):1659–1667.

BHAT: Beta-blockers in Heart Attack Trial. (1990)
Beta-blockers in Heart Attack Trial Investigators. A randomized trial of propranolol in patients with acute myocardial infarction. I. Mortality results. *J. Am. Med. Assoc.* 1982;**247**(12):1707–1714.

BOOST: Bone Marrow Transfer to Enhance ST-Elevation Infarct Regeneration Trial.
Wollert KC, Meyer GP, Lotz J, *et al*. Intracoronary autologous bone marrow cell transfer after myocardial infarction: the BOOST randomized controlled clinical trial. *Lancet* 2004;**364**(9429):141–148.

CAMIAT: Canadian Amiodarone Myocardial Infarction Arrhythmia Trial.
Cairns JA, Connolly SJ, Roberts R, Gent M. Randomized trial of outcome after myocardial infarction in patients with frequent or repetitive ventricular premature depolarizations: CAMIAT. Canadian Amiodarone Myocardial Infarction Arrhythmia Trial Investigators. *Lancet* 1997;**349**(9053):675–682. Erratum in: *Lancet* 1997;**349**(9067):1776.

CAST: Cardiac Arrhythmia Suppression Trial.
Echt DS, Liebson PR, Mitchell LB, et al. Mortality and morbidity in patients receiving encainide, flecainide, or placebo. The Cardiac Arrhythmia Suppression Trial. *N. Engl. J. Med.* 1991;**324**(12):781–788.

CIBIS-II: Cardiac Insufficiency Bisoprolol Study II.
CIBIS-2 Investigators. The Cardiac Insufficiency Bisoprolol Study II (CIBIS-II): a randomized trial. *Lancet* 1999;**353**(9146):9–13.

CCS-1: Chinese Cardiac Study
CCS-1 Investigators. Oral captopril versus placebo among 13,634 patients with suspected acute myocardial infarction: interim report from the Chinese Cardiac Study (CCS-1). *Lancet* 1995;**345**(8951):686–687.

CCS-1 Investigators. Oral captopril versus placebo among 14,962 patients with suspected acute myocardial infarction: a multicenter, randomized, double-blind, placebo controlled clinical trial. Chinese Cardiac Study (CCS-1) Collaborative Group. *Chin. Med. J.* (Engl). 1997;**110**(11):834–838.

CHARM-Added: Candesartan in Heart Failure Assessment of Reduction in Mortality and Morbidity Trial-Added.
McMurray JJ, Ostergren J, Swedberg K, *et al*. CHARM Investigators and Committees. Effects of candesartan in patients with chronic heart failure and reduced left-ventricular systolic function taking angiotensin-converting-enzyme inhibitors: the CHARM-Added trial. *Lancet* 2003;**362**(9386):767–771.

CHARM-Alternative: Candesartan in Heart Failure Assessment of Reduction in Mortality and Morbidity Trial-Alternative.
Granger CB, McMurray JJ, Yusuf S, *et al*. CHARM Investigators and Committees. Effects of candesartan in patients with chronic heart failure and reduced left-ventricular systolic function intolerant to angiotensin-converting-enzyme inhibitors: the CHARM-Alternative trial. *Lancet* 2003;**362**(9386):772–776.

CHARM-Overall: Candesartan in Heart Failure Assessment of Reduction in Mortality and Morbidity Trial-Overall.
Pfeffer MA, Swedberg K, Granger CB, *et al*. CHARM Investigators and Committees. Effects of candesartan on mortality and morbidity in patients with chronic heart failure: the CHARM-Overall programme. *Lancet* 2003;**362**(9386):759–766.

CHARM-Preserved: Candesartan in Heart Failure Assessment of Reduction in Mortality and Morbidity Trial-Preserved.
Yusuf S, Pfeffer MA, Swedberg K, *et al*. CHARM Investigators and Committees. Effects of candesartan in patients with chronic heart failure and preserved left-ventricular ejection fraction: the CHARM-Preserved Trial. *Lancet* 2003;**362**(9386):777–781.

CHF-STAT: Congestive Heart Failure Survival Trial of Antiarrhythmic Therapy.
Singh SN, Fletcher RD, Fisher SG, *et al*. Amiodarone in patients with congestive heart failure and asymptomatic ventricular arrhythmia. Survival Trial of Antiarrhythmic Therapy in Congestive Heart Failure. *N. Engl. J. Med.* 1995;**333**(2):77–82.

CHRISTMAS: Carvedilol Hibernating Reversible Ischaemia Trial.
Cleland JG, Pennell DJ, Ray SG, Coats AJ, Macfarlane PW, Murray GD, Mule JD, Vered Z, Lahiri A; Carvedilol Hibernating Reversible Ischaemia Trial: Marker of success Investigators. Myocardial viability as a determinant of the ejection fraction response to carvedilol in patients with heart failure (CHRISTMAS trial): randomized controlled trial. *Lancet* 2003;**362**(9377):14–21.

COMET: Carvedilol Or Metoprolol European Trial.
Poole-Wilson PA, Swedberg K, Cleland JG, *et al*. Carvedilol Or Metoprolol European Trial Investigators. Comparison of carvedilol and metoprolol on clinical outcomes in patients with chronic heart failure in the Carvedilol Or Metoprolol European Trial (COMET): randomized controlled trial. *Lancet* 2003;**362**(9377):7–13.

COMPANION: Comparison of Medical Therapy, Pacing, and Defibrillation in Chronic Heart Failure.
Bristow MR, Saxon LA, Boehmer J, *et al*. Comparison of Medical Therapy, Pacing, and Defibrillation in Heart Failure (COMPANION) Investigators. Cardiac-resynchronization therapy with or without an implantable defibrillator in advanced chronic heart failure. *N. Engl. J. Med.* 2004;**350**(21):2140–2150.

CONSENSUS: Cooperative North Scandinavian Enalapril Survival Study.
The CONSENSUS Trial Study Group. Effects of enalapril on mortality in severe congestive heart failure. Results of the Cooperative North Scandinavian Enalapril Survival Study (CONSENSUS). *N. Engl. J. Med.* 1987;**316**(23):1429–1435.

COPERNICUS: Carvedilol Prospective Randomized Cumulative Survival Study.
Packer M, Coats AJ, Fowler MB, *et al*. Carvedilol Prospective Randomized Cumulative Survival Study Group. Effect of carvedilol on survival in severe chronic heart failure. *N. Engl. J. Med.* 2001;**344**(22):1651–1658.

DIG: Digitalis Investigation Group.
The Digitalis Investigation Group. The effect of digoxin on mortality and morbidity in patients with heart failure. *N. Engl. J. Med.* 1997;**336**(8):525–533.

ECHOES: Echocardiographic Heart of England Screening Study.
Davies M, Hobbs F, Davis R, *et al*. Prevalence of left-ventricular systolic dysfunction and heart failure in the Echocardiographic Heart of England Screening study: a population based study. *Lancet* 2001;**358**(9280):439–444.

ELITE II: Evaluation of Losartan in the Elderly Trial II.
Pitt B, Poole-Wilson PA, Segal R, *et al*. Effect of losartan compared with captopril on mortality in patients with symptomatic heart failure: randomized trial; the Losartan Heart Failure Survival Study ELITE II. *Lancet* 2000;**355**(9215):1582–1587.

EMIAT: European Amiodarone Myocardial Infarction Arrhythmia Trial.
Julian DG, Camm AJ, Frangin G, *et al*. Randomized trial of effect of amiodarone on mortality in patients with left-ventricular dysfunction after recent myocardial infarction: EMIAT. European Myocardial Infarct Amiodarone Trial Investigators. *Lancet* 1997;**349**(9053):667–674.

EPHESUS: Eplerenone Post-Acute Myocardial Infarction Heart Failure Efficacy and Survival Study.
Pitt B, Remme W, Zannad F, *et al*. Eplerenone Post-Acute Myocardial Infarction Heart Failure Efficacy and Survival Study Investigators. Eplerenone, a selective aldosterone blocker, in patients with left ventricular dysfunction after myocardial infarction. *N. Engl. J. Med.* 2003;**348**(14):1309–1321.

EXPEDITION: Sodium–Proton Exchange Inhibition to Prevent Coronary Events in Acute Cardiac Conditions Trial.
Mentzer RM Jr. Presentation at American Heart Association Scientific Sessions 2003.

Framingham Study:
Ho KK, Pinsky JL, Kannel WB, Levy D. The epidemiology of heart failure: the Framingham Study. *J. Am. Coll. Cardiol.* 1993;**22**(4 Suppl A):6A–13A.

GESICA:
Doval HC, Nul DR, Grancelli HO, Perrone SV, Bortman GR, Curiel R. Randomized trial of low-dose amiodarone in severe congestive heart failure. Grupo de Estudio de la Sobrevida en la Insuficiencia Cardiaca en Argentina (GESICA). *Lancet* 1994;**344**(8921):493–498.

GISSI-3: Gruppo Italiano per lo Studio della Sopravvivenza nell'infarto Miocardico.
GISSI-3 Investigators. GISSI-3: effects of lisinopril and transdermal glyceryl trinitrate singly and together on 6-week mortality and ventricular function after acute myocardial infarction. Gruppo Italiano per lo Studio della Sopravvivenza nell'infarto Miocardico. *Lancet* 1994;**343**(8906):1115–1122.

HOPE: Heart Outcomes Prevention Evaluation.
Yusuf S, Sleight P, Pogue J, Bosch J, Davies R, Dagenais G. Effects of an angiotensin-converting enzyme inhibitor, ramipril, on cardiovascular events in high-risk patients. The Heart Outcomes Prevention Evaluation Study Investigators. *N. Engl. J. Med.* 2000;**342**(3):145–153. Erratum in: *N. Engl. J. Med.* 2000;**342**(18):1376; *N. Engl. J. Med.* 2000;**342**(10):748.

IONA: Impact of Nicorandil in Angina.
IONA Study group. Effect of nicorandil on coronary events in patients with stable angina: the Impact Of Nicorandil in Angina (IONA) randomized trial. *Lancet* 2002;**359**(9314):1269–1275. Erratum in: *Lancet* 2002;**360**(9335):806.

ISIS-4: Fourth International Study of Infarct Survival
ISIS-4 (Fourth International Study of Infarct Survival) Collaborative Group. ISIS-4: a randomized factorial trial assessing early oral captopril, oral mononitrate, and intravenous magnesium sulphate in 58,050 patients with suspected acute myocardial infarction. *Lancet* 1995;**345**(8951):669–685.

LIDO: Levosimendan Infusion versus DObutamine in severe congestive heart failure.
Follath F, Cleland JGF, Just H, *et al*. Efficacy and safety of intravenous levosimendan compared with dobutamine in severe low-output heart failure (the LIDO study): a randomized double-blind trial. *Lancet* 2002;**360**:196–202.

MDC: Metoprolol in Dilated Cardiomyopathy Study.
Metoprolol in Dilated Cardiomyopathy (MDC) Trial Study Group. Beneficial effect of metoprolol in idiopathic dilated cardiomyopathy. *Lancet* 1993;**342**:1441–1446.

MERIT-HF: Metoprolol CR/XL Randomized Intervention Trial in Congestive Heart Failure.
MERIT-HF Investigators. Effect of metoprolol CR/XL in chronic heart failure: Metoprolol CR/XL Randomized Intervention Trial in Congestive Heart Failure (MERIT-HF). *Lancet* 1999;**353**(9169):2001–2007.

Minnesota Living with Heart Failure Questionnaire.
Rector TS, Cohn JN. Assessment of patient outcome with the Minnesota Living with Heart Failure questionnaire: reliability and validity during a randomized, double-blind, placebo-controlled trial of pimobendan. Pimobendan Multicenter Research Group. *Am. Heart J.* 1992;**124**(4):1017–1025.

MONICA: MONitoring trends and determinants in CArdiovascular disease.
McDonagh TA, Morrison CE, Lawrence A, *et al.* Symptomatic and asymptomatic LVSD in an urban population. *Lancet* 1997;**350**:829–833.

PRAISE: Prospective Randomized Amlodipine Survival Evaluation.
Packer M, O'Connor CM, Ghali JK, *et al.* for the Prospective Randomized Amlodipine Survival Evaluation Study Group. Effect of amlodipine on morbidity in severe chronic heart failure. *N. Engl. J. Med.* 1996;**335**(15):1107–1114.

PRIME II: Second Prospective Randomized Study of Ibopamine on Mortality and Efficacy.
Hampton JR, van Veldhuisen DJ, Kleber FX, *et al.* Randomized study of effect of ibopamine on survival in patients with advanced severe heart failure. Second Prospective Randomized Study of Ibopamine on Mortality and Efficacy (PRIME II) Investigators. *Lancet* 1997;**349**(9057):971–977.

PROMISE: Prospective Randomized Milrinone Survival Evaluation.
Packer M, Carver JR, Rodeheffer RJ, *et al.* Effect of oral milrinone on mortality in severe chronic heart failure. The PROMISE Study Research Group. *N. Engl. J. Med.* 1991;**325**(21):1468–1475.

PROVED: Prospective Randomized study Of Ventricular failure and the Efficacy of Digoxin.
Uretsky BF, Young JB, Shahidi FE, Yellen LG, Harrison MC, Jolly MK. Randomized study assessing the effect of digoxin withdrawal in patients with mild to moderate chronic congestive heart failure: results of the PROVED trial. PROVED Investigative Group. *J. Am. Coll. Cardiol.* 1993;**22**(4):955–962.

Quinapril Heart Failure Trial.
Pflugfelder PW, Baird MG, Tonkon MJ, DiBianco R, Pitt B. Clinical consequences of angiotensin-converting enzyme inhibitor withdrawal in chronic heart failure: a double-blind, placebo-controlled study of quinapril. The Quinapril Heart Failure Trial Investigators. *J. Am. Coll. Cardiol.* 1993;**22**(6):1557–1563.

RADIANCE: Randomized Assessment of Digoxin on Inhibitors of the ANgiotensin Converting Enzyme.
Packer M, Gheorghiade M, Young JB, *et al.* Withdrawal of digoxin from patients with chronic heart failure treated with angiotensin-converting enzyme inhibitors. RADIANCE Study. *N. Engl. J. Med.* 1993;**329**(1):1–7.

RALES: Randomized Aldactone Evaluation Study.
Pitt B, Zannad F, Remme WJ, *et al.* The effect of spironolactone on morbidity and mortality in patients with severe heart failure. Randomized Aldactone Evaluation Study Investigators. *N. Engl. J. Med.* 1999;**341**(10):709–717.

RESTOR-MV: Randomized Evaluation of a Surgical Treatment for Off-pump Repair of the Mitral Valve. Trial in progress.

SAVE: Survival and Ventricular Enlargement Trial.
Pfeffer MA, Braunwald E, Moye LA, *et al.* Effect of captopril on mortality and morbidity in patients with left ventricular dysfunction after myocardial infarction. Results of the survival and ventricular enlargement trial. The SAVE Investigators. *N. Engl. J. Med.* 1992;**327**(10):669–677.

SCD-HeFT: Sudden Cardiac Death in Heart Failure Trial.
Cleland JG, Ghosh J, Freemantle N, *et al.* Clinical trials update and cumulative meta-analyses from the American College of Cardiology: WATCH, SCD-HeFT, DINAMIT, CASINO, INSPIRE, STRATUS-US, RIO-Lipids and cardiac resynchronization therapy in heart failure. *Eur. J. Heart Fail.* 2004;**6**(4):501–508.

SHOCK: Should we Emergently Revascularize Occluded Coronaries for Cardiogenic Shock Trial.
Hochman JS, Sleeper LA, Webb JG, *et al*. Early revascularization in acute myocardial infarction complicated by cardiogenic shock. SHOCK Investigators. Should We Emergently Revascularize Occluded Coronaries for Cardiogenic Shock. *N. Engl. J. Med.* 1999;**341**(9):625–634.

SMILE: Survival of Myocardial Infarction Long-Term Evaluation.
Ambrosioni E, Borghi C, Magnani B. The effect of the angiotensin-converting-enzyme inhibitor zofenopril on mortality and morbidity after anterior myocardial infarction. The Survival of Myocardial Infarction Long-Term Evaluation (SMILE) Study Investigators. *N. Engl. J. Med.* 1995;**332**(2):80–85.

SOLVD: Studies of Left Ventricular Dysfunction (1997); *Am. J. Cardiol.* 79:909–.
Dries DL, Domanski MJ, Waclawiw MA, Gersh BJ. Effect of antithrombotic therapy on risk of sudden coronary death in patients with congestive heart failure. *Am. J. Cardiol.* 1997;**79**(7):909–913.
The SOLVD Investigators. Effect of enalapril on mortality and the development of heart failure in asymptomatic patients with reduced left ventricular ejection fractions. *N. Engl. J. Med.* 1992;**327**(10):685–691. Erratum in: *N. Engl. J. Med.* 1992;**327**(24):1768.

SOLVD-T: Studies of Left Ventricular Dysfunction-Treatment Trial.
The SOLVD Investigators. Effects of enalapril on survival in patients with reduced left ventricular ejection fractions and congestive heart failure. *N. Engl. J. Med.* 1991;**325**:293–302.

SPAF: Stroke Prevention in Atrial Fibrillation.
The Stroke Prevention in Atrial Fibrillation Investigators. Predictors of thromboembolism in atrial fibrillation: I. Clinical features of patients at risk. *Ann. Intern. Med.* 1992;**116**(1):1–5.
The Stroke Prevention in Atrial Fibrillation Investigators. Predictors of thromboembolism in atrial fibrillation: II. Echocardiographic features of patients at risk. The Stroke Prevention in Atrial Fibrillation Investigators. *Ann. Intern. Med.* 1992;**116**(1):6–12.

SPORTIF III:
Olsson SB. Executive Steering Committee on behalf of SPORTIF III Investigators. Stroke prevention with the oral direct thrombin inhibitor ximelagatran compared with warfarin in patients with nonvalvular atrial fibrillation. *Lancet* 2003;**362**:1691–1698.

STRETCH: Symptom Tolerability Response to Exercise Trial of Candesartan Cilexitil in Heart Failure Trial.
Riegger GA, Bouzo H, Petr P, *et al*. Improvement in exercise tolerance and symptoms of congestive heart failure during treatment with candesartan cilexetil. Symptom, Tolerability, Response to Exercise Trial of Candesartan Cilexetil in Heart Failure (STRETCH) Investigators. *Circulation* 1999;**100**(22):2224–2230.

TORIC: TOrasemide In Congestive Heart Failure.
Cosin J, Diez J; TORIC investigators. Torasemide in chronic heart failure: results of the TORIC study. *Eur. J. Heart Fail.* 2002;**4**(4):507–513. Erratum in: *Eur. J. Heart Fail* 2002;**4**(5):667.

TRACE: Trandalopril Cardiac Evaluation.
Kober L, Torp-Pedersen C, Carlsen JE, *et al*. A clinical trial of the angiotensin-converting enzyme inhibitor trandolapril in patients with left ventricular dysfunction after myocardial infarction. Trandolapril Cardiac Evaluation (TRACE) Study Group. *N. Engl. J. Med.* 1995;**333**(25):1670–1676.
Torp-Pedersen C, Kober L. Effect of ACE inhibitor trandolapril on life expectancy of patients with reduced left-ventricular function after acute myocardial infarction. TRACE Study Group. Trandolapril Cardiac Evaluation. *Lancet* 1999;**354**(9172):9–12.

UK-HEART: UK Heart Failure Evaulation and Assessment of Risk Trial.
Nolan J, Batin PD, Andrews R, *et al*. Prospective study of heart rate variability and mortality in chronic heart failure: results of the UK Heart Failure Evaluation and Assessment of Risk Trial. *Circulation* 1998;**98**(15):1510–1516.

US Carvedilol Heart Failure Study.
Colucci WS, Packer M, Bristow MR, *et al*. Carvedilol inhibits clinical progression in patients with mild symptoms of heart failure. US Carvedilol Heart Failure Study Group. *Circulation* 1996;**94**(11):2800–2806.

USCT: US Carvedilol Trial.
Packer M, Bristow MR, Cohn JN, *et al*. The effect of carvedilol on morbidity and mortality in patients with chronic heart failure. US Carvedilol Heart Failure Study Group. *N. Engl. J. Med.* 1996;**334**:1349–1355.

VHeFT-I, -II: Vasodilators in Heart Failure Trial I, II.
Cohn JN, Archibald DG, Ziesche S, *et al*. Effect of vasodilator therapy on mortality in chronic congestive heart failure. Results of a Veterans Administration Cooperative Study. *N.Engl. J. Med.* 1986;**314**:1547–1552.
Cohn JN, Johnson G, Ziesche S, *et al*. A comparison of enalapril with hydralazine-isosorbide dinitrate in the treatment of chronic congestive heart failure. *N. Engl. J. Med.* 1991;**325**:303–310.

ValHeFT: Valsartan Heart Failure Trial.
Cohn JN, Tognoni G; Valsartan Heart Failure Trial Investigators. A randomized trial of the angiotensin-receptor blocker valsartan in chronic heart failure. *N. Engl. J. Med.* 2001;**345**(23):1667–1675.

VALIANT: Valsartan in Acute Myocardial Infarction Trial.
Pfeffer MA, McMurray JJ, Velazquez EJ, *et al*. Valsartan in Acute Myocardial Infarction Trial Investigators. Valsartan, captopril, or both in myocardial infarction complicated by heart failure, left ventricular dysfunction, or both. *N. Engl. J. Med.* 2003;**349**(20):1893–1906. Epub 2003 Nov 10.

VEST: Vesnarinone Trial.
Cohn JN, Goldstein SO, Greenberg BH, *et al*. A dose-dependent increase in mortality with vesnarinone among patients with severe heart failure. Vesnarinone Trial Investigators. *N. Engl. J. Med.* 1998;**339**:1810–1816.

WARCEF: Warfarin Aspirin Reduced Cardiac Ejection Fraction Study.
Cleland JG, Ghosh J, Freemantle N, *et al*. Clinical trials update and cumulative meta-analyses from the American College of Cardiology: WATCH, SCD-HeFT, DINAMIT, CASINO, INSPIRE, STRATUS-US, RIO-Lipids and cardiac resynchronization therapy in heart failure. *Eur. J. Heart Fail.* 2004;**6**(4):501–508.

WATCH: Warfarin and Antiplatelet Therapy in Chronic Heart Failure.
Cleland JG, Ghosh J, Freemantle N, *et al*. Clinical trials update and cumulative meta-analyses from the American College of Cardiology: WATCH, SCD-HeFT, DINAMIT, CASINO, INSPIRE, STRATUS-US, RIO-Lipids and cardiac resynchronization therapy in heart failure. *Eur. J. Heart Fail.* 2004;**6**(4):501–508.

APPENDIX B
WEBSITES
Abiomed Inc: http://www.abiomed.com
American College of Cardiology: http://www.acc.org
American Heart Association: http://www.aha.org
American Society of Hypertension: http://ash-us.org
Blood Pressure Association: http://www.bpassoc.org.uk
British Cardiac Society: http://www.bcs.com
British Heart Foundation: http://www.bhf.org.uk
British Hypertension Society: http://www.bhsoc.org
British Society of Echocardiography: http://www.bcs.com/affiliates/bse/html
Cardiomyopathy Association: http://www.cardiomyopathy.org
Coronary Prevention Group: http://www.healthnet.org.uk
European Atherosclerosis Society: http://www.eas-society.org
European Heart Network: http://www.ehnheart.org
European Society of Cardiology: http://escardio.org
European Society of Hypertension: http://www.eshonline.org
Heart Failure Society of America: http://www.hfsa.org
Heart UK: http://www.heratuk.org.uk
National Heart Forum: http://www.heartforum.org.uk
National Heart Lung and Blood Institute: http://nhi.org
Primary Care Cardiovascular Society: http://www.pccs.org.uk
Syncardia Systems Inc: http://www.syncardia.com

APPENDIX C
CLASSIFICATIONS AND GUIDELINES
New York Heart Association Classification

- Class I: Asymptomatic. No limitation of exercise capacity, but evidence of cardiac dysfunction on e.g. echocardiography.
- Class II: Mild. Slight limitation of exercise capacity, with symptoms on significant exertion e.g. walking up several flights of stairs.
- Class III: Moderate. Significant limitation of activities; symptoms on mild exertion but not at rest.
- Class IV: Severe. Severely limited; symptoms at rest.

Recommendations for diagnosis of heart failure (UK National Institute for Clinical Excellence)

Suspected heart failure because of history, symptoms, and signs.

Seek to exclude heart failure through:
- 12-lead ECG;
- and/or natriuretic peptides (BNP or NTproBNP) – where available.

Other recommended tests (mostly to exclude other conditions):
- Chest X-ray.
- Blood tests: U&Es, creatinine, FBC, TFTs, LFTs, glucose, and lipids.
- Urinalysis, peak flow or spirometry.

Both ECG and natriuretic peptides – normal heart failure unlikely; consider alternative diagnosis.

One or more abnormal
↓
Imaging by echocardiography

No abnormality detected
Heart failure unlikely, but if diagnostic doubt persists consider diastolic dysfunction and consider referral for specialist assessment.

Abnormal
- Assess heart failure severity, aetiology, precipitating and exacerbating factors and type of cardiac dysfunction.
- Correctable causes must be identified.
- Consider referral.

BNP: brain natriuretic protein; ECG: electrocardiogram; FBC: full blood count; LFT: liver function test; TFT: thyroid function test; U&E: urine and electrolytes.

UK NICE recommendations for cardiac resynchronization therapy

CRT should be considered in selected patients with:
- LV systolic dysfunction (LVEF ≤35%).
- Drug refractory symptoms.
- QRS duration >120 ms.

The results of ongoing trials will help to guide appropriate patient selection. CRT: cardiac resynchronization therapy; LV: left ventricular; LVEF: left ventricular ejection fraction; NICE: National Institute for Clinical Excellence.

UK NICE recommendations for implantable cardioverter defibrillators

ICD use should be routinely considered for patients in the following categories:

Secondary prevention, i.e. for patients who present, in the absence of a treatable cause with:
- Cardiac arrest due to either VT or VF.
- Spontaneous sustained VT causing syncope or significant haemodynamic compromise.
- Sustained VT without syncope/cardiac arrest and who have an associated reduction in EF (<35%) but are no worse than NYHA III.

Primary prevention for patients with:
- A history of previous MI and all of the following:
- Nonsustained VT on Holter 24-hour ECG.
- Inducible VT on electrophysiological testing.
- LV dysfunction with an EF <35% and are no worse than NYHA III.
- A familial cardiac condition with a high risk of sudden death including long QT syndrome, hypertrophic cardiomyopathy, Brugada syndrome, arrhythmogenic right ventricular dysplasia, and following repair of tetralogy of Fallot.

ECG: electrocardiogram; EF: ejection fraction; ICD: implantable cardioverter defibrillator; LV: left ventricular; MI: myocardial infarction; NICE: National Institute for Clinical Excellence; NYHA: New York Heart Association; VF: ventricular fibrillation; VT: ventricular tachycardia.

APPENDIX D DRUGS USED IN HEART FAILURE

	Example	Preparation	Initial daily dose	Maintenance daily dose (maximum)	Common side-effects
Angiotensin-converting enzyme inhibitors					
Captopril	Acepril	Oral	6.25–12.5 bd/tds	25 mg bd/tds	Cough, hypotension, rash, raised urea, creatinine, potassium, upper respiratory tract effects, gastro-intestinal effects, liver function abnormalities, angioedema, headache, myalgia
	Capoten	Oral	6.25–12.5 mg	25 mg bd/tds (150 mg)	
Cilazapril	Vascace	Oral	500 µg	1–2.5 mg (5 mg)	
Enalapril	Innovace	Oral	2.5 mg	20 mg in 1–2 divided doses	
Fosinopril	Staril	Oral	10 mg	40 mg (40 mg)	
Lisinopril	Carace	Oral	2.5 mg	5–20 mg	
	Zestril	Oral	2.5 mg	5–20 mg	
Perindopril	Coversyl	Oral	2 mg	4 mg	
Quinapril	Accupro	Oral	2.5 mg	10–20 mg (40 mg)	
Ramipril	Tritace	Oral	1.25 mg	10 mg (10 mg)	
Trandolapril	Gopten	Oral	UL		
	Odrik	Oral	UL		
Angiotensin receptor blockers					
Candesartan	Amias	Oral	4 mg	Titrate doubling at 2 week intervals (32 mg)	All of ACE inhibitor side-effects except cough
Eprosartan	Teveten	Oral	UL		
Irbesartan	Aprovel	Oral	UL		
Losartan	Cozaar	Oral	UL		
Telmisartan	Micardis	Oral	UL		
Valsartan	Diovan	Oral	UL	Titrate up over several weeks (160 mg bd)	
Cardiac glycosides					
Digoxin	Lanoxin	Oral/IV		62.5–250 µg	Nausea, xanthopsia, arrhythmia
Beta-blockers – titrate up slowly to maximum tolerated dose					
Bisoprolol	Cardicor	Oral	1.25 mg od	10.0 mg	Peripheral vasoconstriction, conduction disorders, bradycardia
	Emcor	Oral	1.25 mg od	10.0 mg	
	Monocor	Oral	1.25 mg od	10.0 mg	
Carvedilol	Eucardic	Oral	3.125 mg bd	25 mg bd (50 mg bd if weight >85 kg)	
Metoprolol (immediate release)	Metoprolol Tartrate	Oral	5 mg bd*	50 mg bd*	
	Lopresor/Betaloc	Oral	UL		

Drug	Brand	Route	Dose	Dose	Side effects
Metoprolol (CR/XL)	Metoprolol Succinate	Oral	25 mg od**	200 mg od**	
Diuretics *Loop diuretics*					Hyponatraemia, hypokalaemia, hypomagnesaemia, hypercalcaemia, gout, ototoxicity, myalgia
Bumetanide (Bumetadine)	Burinex	Oral/IV	1.0 mg	5 mg	
Furosemide (Frusemide)	Lasix	Oral/IV	40–80 mg		
Torasemide (Torsemide)	Torem	Oral/IV	5 mg	20 mg (40 mg)	
Potassium-sparing diuretics/Aldosterone antagonists					Hyperkalaemia, hypotension, renal dysfunction
Amiloride	Generic	Oral	5 mg	20 mg	
Spironolactone	Aldactone	Oral	12.5–25 mg	2.5 mg (50 mg)	Gynaecomastia
Eplerenone	Inspra	Oral	25 mg	50 mg (only licensed for post-MI)	
Triamterene	Dytac	Oral	25–50 mg	100–200 mg	
Thiazide diuretics and related compounds					Postural hypotension, hyponatraemia, hypokalaemia, hypomagnesaemia, hypochloraemia, hypocalcaemia, alkalosis, hyperuricaemia, hyperglycaemia
Bendroflumethiazide	Neo-Naclex	Oral	2.5 mg	2.5 mg	
Chlorthalidone (Chlortalidone)	Hygroton	Oral	25–50 mg	100–200 mg	
Cyclopenthiazide	Navidrex	Oral	250–500 µg	1 mg	
Indapamide	Natrilix	Oral	2.5 mg	2.5 mg	
Metolazone	Metenix 5	Oral	2.5 mg	10 mg	
Xipamide	Diurexan	Tablet 20 mg	40–80 mg	20 mg *in combination with loop diuretic e.g. 2.5 mg weekly*	
Nitrates and related compounds					Injection: severe hypotension, nausea, palpitations; all formulations: throbbing headache, flushing, dizziness, postural hypotension, tachycardia
Glyceryl trinitrate	Nitrocine Suscard Buccal Bidil	IV infusion Buccal Oral	Titrate to symptoms 5 mg tds UL	10 mg tds UL	
Hydralazine/isosorbide dinitrate					
Levosimendan	Simdax	IV bolus/ infusion	6–12 µg	0.05–0.2 µg/kg/min	Headache, hypotension

	Example	Preparation	Initial daily dose	Maintenance daily dose (maximum)	Common side-effects
Phosphodiesterase inhibitors					
Enoximone	Perfan	IV infusion	0.5–1 mg or 90 µg/min	500 µg/30 min (3 mg/kg 3–6 hr) 5–20 µg/kg/min (24 mg/kg)	Ectopic beats, ventricular tachycardia or supraventricular arrhythmia, hypotension, headache, nausea
Milrinone	Primacor	IV infusion	50 µg/kg	375–750 µg/kg/min for 48–72 hr (1.13 mg/kg)	
Vesnarinone					
Calcium channel blockers *Dihydropyridines*					Headache, flushing, dizziness
Amlodipine	Istin	Oral	5 mg	5 mg (10 mg)	
Felodipine	Plendil	Oral	5 mg	5 mg (10 mg)	
Antiarrhythmics					
Amiodarone	Cordarone	Oral/IV	200 mg tds	100–200 mg	Pigmentation, photosensitivy, grey skin, pulmonary fibrosis, corneal microdeposits, peripheral neuropathy, hypo-/hyperthy-roidism, abnormal liver function, prolonged QT interval, torsades de pointes
Dofetilide		Oral	500 µg bd		Prolonged QT interval, torsades de pointes
Sympathomimetics					
Beta-1 Dobutamine	Posiject	IV infusion	2.5–10 µg/kg/min		Tachycardia, hypotension
Mixed Dopamine	Generic	IV infusion	2–5 µg/kg/min		Nausea, vomiting, peripheral vasoconstriction, tachycardia
Antithrombotics					
Aspirin	Generic	Oral	Dose dependent on indication, not yet of proven value in HF		Bleeds, gastrointestinal upset
Clopidogrel	Plavix	Oral	"		Bleeding, rashes
Warfarin	Marevan	Oral	"		Bleeding
Ximelagatran		Oral			Abnormal liver function, bleeding

UL: unlicensed   *These are the doses used in the COMET trial; Metoprolol is not licensed for use in heart failure in the UK
**These are the doses used in the MERIT-HF trial; Metoprolol is not licensed for use in heart failure in the UK

Index

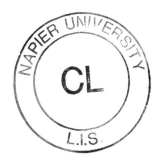